UNDERSTANDING
MENTAL
ILLNESS

UNDERSTANDING
MENTAL
ILLNESS

A Comprehensive Guide to Mental Health Disorders for Family and Friends

Carlin Barnes, MD, and
Marketa Wills, MD, MBA

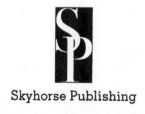

Skyhorse Publishing

Skyhorse Publishing books may be purchased in bulk at special discounts for sales promotion, corporate gifts, fund-raising, or educational purposes. Special editions can also be created to specifications. For details, contact the Special Sales Department, Skyhorse Publishing, 307 West 36th Street, 11th Floor, New York, NY 10018 or info@skyhorsepublishing.com.

Skyhorse® and Skyhorse Publishing® are registered trademarks of Skyhorse Publishing, Inc.®, a Delaware corporation.

Visit our website at www.skyhorsepublishing.com.

10 9 8 7 6 5 4 3 2 1

Library of Congress Control Number: 2019944853

Cover design by Daniel Brount
Cover image: Gettyimages

Print ISBN: 978-1-5107-4594-0
Ebook ISBN: 978-1-5107-4596-4

Printed in the United States of America

Contents

Contents

Introduction

EVERYONE HAS A STORY, INCLUDING the reason (or reasons) why that person chooses their occupation. Sometimes it's for money; sometimes it's for recognition. Often, people do what they do because it gives them a great sense of self-fulfillment—a feeling that they are achieving what they were put on Earth to accomplish. Many enter a particular profession because it's the best way they know how to give something back to a community in which they have some sort of vested interest.

Practitioners in the field of psychiatry run this full gamut of reasons. But there are also a number of other prevalent factors that you will see in most behavioral health professionals. First and foremost, we believe, is an innate sense of curiosity about humanity as a whole—and on a more micro level, about each individual human being. What makes people behave as they do? What makes them tick? This is part of the foundation of psychiatry: a driving inquisitiveness through which we are afforded the opportunity to tap into another person's thoughts, feelings, and experiences in order to help that person live a more whole and fulfilling life.

The next factor is an overwhelming desire to connect with people on a very real and personal level. This is not for any sort of personal gain, but to help them, in turn, connect more fully with themselves as well as with their families, friends, employers, coworkers, and so on. While mental health begins with an individual, it has the potential to affect everyone in that person's life and the relationships between them, so the approach to treatment must be holistic.

The list of characteristics of those in the psychiatric field could go on and on. It is complex work. This business of dealing with other people's thoughts and feelings, and how those thoughts and feelings are influenced by the chemical makeup of their brains, can be complicated. It takes a certain sort of individual to pursue this line of work. So, why do we do what we do? And what makes us think it's so important? Allow us to introduce ourselves by way of an explanation and to tell you a little about our purpose in writing this book—and why we believe you should read it.

Dr. Carlin Barnes

For as long as I can remember, I have always been interested in the *why* of human behaviors, and I can trace this back to a very specific time in my life that put those wheels in motion. When I was about five years old, my aunt and uncle, both alcoholics, got into a brawl that turned violent. She ended up killing him and going to prison. In her absence, and with her husband gone, there was no one to care for their ten children, so they were sent to live with various family members. My little family—just my parents and me at the time—took in my twin cousins, both of whom suffered from several emotional problems, including speech delays, undiagnosed ADHD, and severe anxiety symptoms. My parents did the best they could for them, even seeking professional psychiatric help and getting them on psychotropic medications. None of this was discussed openly. The entire process was quite secretive; mental illness, in my family as in so many others, was seen as a shameful condition and something to be minimized, denied, or shunned.

Yet it affected all of us. My father worked long hours to support us all, and my mother was overburdened by the enormous task of caring for my cousins because of their special emotional needs. In turn, I was put in a sort of parental role, filling in where my parents, for reasons they could not entirely control, fell short. It was a difficult time, a hardship for us all precipitated by my cousins' behaviors. This time in my life was the catalyst for my interest in human behaviors and the impact of mental illness on individuals and families. I saw and experienced firsthand the devastating impact that illnesses such as alcoholism and mood disorders can have on one's life—not only for the individual, but for everyone the individual loves.

Though there have been additional highlights in my life that have led me to my love for the field of psychiatry, this introduction to mental illness at a young and impressionable age had the most significant impact. Due, I believe, to those early experiences, I went into medicine with the intent not just to treat patients, but to really listen to them and develop beneficial, therapeutic relationships with them. Toward this end, I have amassed a wealth of clinical experience. The groundwork for my current clinical practice was laid as I graduated from some of the finest institutions and programs in the country. I have a BA in psychology with a focus on premed studies from the University of Virginia, and I attended the Texas A&M College of Medicine, graduating with an MD. I completed a residency in adult psychiatry at the Cambridge Hospital, a Harvard Medical School-affiliated program. I also completed a fellowship in child and adolescent psychiatry at Emory University School of Medicine. I am certified by the American Board of Psychiatry and Neurology in both adult psychiatry and child and adolescent psychiatry, and I am a member of the American Academy of Child and Adolescent Psychiatry, the National Medical Association, and the Black Psychiatrists of America.

Currently, I have fifteen years of clinical posttraining practice experience. I've practiced in several community mental health center settings in Texas and Georgia and provided psychiatric services within the juvenile forensic system. I've been in private practice since 2008 in Houston, working with children, adolescents, and adults. I commonly see and treat a myriad of psychiatric conditions, including ADHD, depressive disorders, anxiety disorders, autism spectrum disorders, and adjustment disorders. Recently, I have stepped into the position of a behavioral health medical director at a Fortune 500 managed-care insurance company. Due to my passion for this field, I often speak on mental health topics at community and civic organizations and events such as church groups, sorority events, and community forums.

Dr. Marketa Wills

As a student in medical school, I worked with many different kinds of patients. The purpose of these rotations is to help the student choose which field of medicine they would like to enter. For me, at the end of it all, it came down to two choices—emergency medicine or psychiatry—the two areas that I had found suited me the most. I liked the immediacy of working in the emergency room and the variety of issues and illnesses I got to treat; there was never a boring minute, and I learned something new every day.

At the same time, though, I appreciated the slower nature of the psychiatric field, where the doctor-patient relationship extends over longer periods of time. I was also intensely interested in how psychiatry would allow me to see deep into people's lives in a very impactful way in order to help them discover more about themselves. Psychiatry is all about self-discovery and believing that we all can be different and better human beings, and it's a wonder and a privilege to be able to help people through the stages that will get them to that fully realized place.

In the end, believe it or not, I made my decision based on the clock. I realized that when I worked in the emergency room and I glanced at the clock, I was subconsciously calculating how much longer it would be until my shift would end. With psychiatry, however, when I glanced at the clock, it was always much later than I'd thought it would be. I became so absorbed in my work that I didn't even notice how quickly the hours had passed. This, I thought, had to be a sign that psychiatry was my calling in life.

By the time I chose this path, I had already completed my undergraduate years at Brown University in Providence, Rhode Island, majoring in sociology and premed, and I was obtaining my MD at the University of Pennsylvania School of Medicine. I completed my residency in psychiatry at Massachusetts General Hospital and McLean Hospital, both of which are premier teaching institutions affiliated with Harvard Medical School. I also earned an MBA in health-care management and finance from the world-renowned Wharton School in Philadelphia, and I am certified in adult psychiatry by the American Board of Psychiatry and Neurology.

Since graduating from residency, my career has been a sort of hybrid between direct patient care and executive leadership. I worked at McKinsey & Company as a health-care consultant and was the director of physician affairs at a large teaching hospital in Texas. I've been the medical director of a women's behavioral unit, where I focused on women with acute perinatal and postpartum psychiatric issues, and I've also followed indigent patients in an outpatient community mental health setting. Since 2012, I have been a medical director in a Fortune 500 managed-care setting. I have served in many leadership roles in various professional, civic, and philanthropic organizations. As a community servant-leader, I am often asked to speak on mental health topics, and I enjoy educating those in my community on how to lead their best lives. Recently, I was appointed to the board of the National Alliance on Mental Illness, Hillsborough County, Florida.

How We Came Together, and the Pact

Some things are destined to be. Our meeting, bonding, and coming together to form a pact with this project is a perfect example. Our lives and interests, both professional and personal, parallel each other's in many areas. We both are passionate about delivering quality mental health care and ensuring the widest possible access. It is this passion that motivates us to educate others about psychiatric conditions. Personally, our lives' paths have brought us together through a series of events and experiences. We first met while working together for a health-care company over a two-year period. It was then we realized our common interests and histories. In addition to both being female psychiatrists, we both attended residency programs affiliated with Harvard Medical School. Through conversation, we learned that we share a passion for the arts and a call to serve the community, and in fact, we belong to the same sorority. Naturally, we both belong to many of the same professional and social organizations. One might even say that we share both a professional and personal sisterhood!

With this in mind, it is not surprising we both wanted to work on a project to help educate people about psychiatric disorders and the effective interventions available. What began as an organic conversation about reaching people with more detailed mental health information gradually transformed into this book. Both of us had experienced the abundance of misinformation surrounding psychiatric conditions among the public. In many instances, this served as an obstacle to individuals seeking and receiving effective therapy. Thus, we formed a pact to create an educational platform that would reach beyond our local spheres of influence. This book serves as our initial effort to get accurate information about the most common mental health conditions people experience today to those who need it.

Why Read This Book?

Many of our families have someone—a brother, a sister, an aunt, an uncle, a cousin—who seems to behave a little differently from everyone else. Maybe they always seem to be saying the wrong thing at the wrong time, embarrassing you in front of other family members or friends. Maybe they all too often seem despondent, sad, and withdrawn, unable to cope with everyday life. If a child, their constant hyperactivity makes them a real handful to deal with and interferes with everyday activities at school and home.

What may someone suffering from a mental illness look like? They may have thoughts or behaviors that appear out of touch with reality. They may be engaging in very impulsive, risky, or dangerous acts. There may be an addiction to drugs or alcohol. These are just a few examples. The list of possible behaviors and symptoms is unfortunately long.

There are myriad ways in which individuals with mental illnesses, diagnosed or not, can affect those who love and care for them. And there are just as many ways in which we can react to their behaviors. We can call them quirky or odd and leave it at that. We can place blame or be judgmental. We can run ourselves ragged trying to find a "cure" for what ails them or making excuses for their behaviors.

Oftentimes we take the path of least resistance—we simply ignore the problem and hope that it goes away. This is a route frequently taken due to the stigma of mental illness in our society. Many would rather let their loved ones go untreated than admit they might have a mental illness. But where does this get them in the end? People with untreated mental illnesses make up one third of the nation's homeless population and 16 percent of inmates in our jails and prisons. They are more likely to be victimized—robbed, raped, even murdered—and the crimes against them largely go unreported, because who would believe them anyway?[1]

On the other hand, a Department of Justice study found that 4.3 percent of homicides were committed by people with histories of untreated mental illness, and a MacArthur Foundation study found that individuals with mental illness committed twice as many violent acts just prior to being admitted to hospitals and during periods when they were unmedicated. Posthospitalization, the study showed that rate dropped by 50 percent.[2] Still, up to 54 percent of individuals with serious mental illnesses receive no treatment[3]; of those who do receive treatment, 46 percent are off their medications only nine months later.[4]

What does this mean in the big picture? The longer a person with a mental illness goes untreated, the less able they may be to achieve any

---

1 Sentencing Project (US). Mentally ill offenders in the criminal justice system: An analysis and prescription. Washington D.C.: Sentencing Project, 2002. Retrieved from https://www.sentencingproject.org/wp-content/uploads/2016/01/Mentally-Ill-Offenders-in-the-Criminal-Justice-System.pdf.

2 Steadman, Henry J., Edward P. Mulvey, John Monahan, Pamela Clark Robbins, Paul S. Appelbaum, Thomas Grisso, Loren H. Roth, and Eric Silver. "Violence by people discharged from acute psychiatric inpatient facilities and by others in the same neighborhoods." Archives of general psychiatry 55, no. 5 (1998): 393–401.

3 Kessler, Ronald C., Patricia A. Berglund, Martha L. Bruce, J. Randy Koch, Eugene M. Laska, Philip J. Leaf, Ronald W. Manderscheid, Robert A. Rosenheck, Ellen E. Walters, and Philip S. Wang. "The prevalence and correlates of untreated serious mental illness." Health services research 36, no. 6 Pt 1 (2001): 987–1007.

4 Vanelli, Mark, Philip Burstein, and Joyce Cramer. "Refill patterns of atypical and conventional antipsychotic medications at a national retail pharmacy chain." Psychiatric Services 52, no. 9 (2001): 1248–1250.

sort of long-term recovery. Study after study has shown that the longer one waits to begin treatment, the greater the severity of the mental illness becomes, and the more difficult it becomes to combat. Conversely, early treatment consistently leads to much more positive outcomes.

These statistics and facts paint a bleak picture—but this is where you come in. Knowledge is power. Being aware and informed is the first step in helping a loved one or family member get the proper treatment they need to begin the road to recovery and emotional wellness. Armed with the knowledge of clear and factual information, you will be able to begin the process of helping your loved one. Change will not happen overnight; recovery is a process that is a different journey for each person. The most important thing is that you all hang in there—that you let your loved one know that you are with them for the long haul, through the good and the bad, no matter what the outcome. Our goal is that this book will give you the reassurance and information you need to do just that.

Disclaimer: The information and materials in this book are provided with the intent to inform, educate, and enhance awareness regarding common mental health issues. This book and its contents, however, are not intended to replace professional mental health diagnosis, evaluation, care, and/or treatment. Likewise, this book and its contents should not be used for the purposes of self-diagnosis and/or self-treatment.

Chapter 1
What Is Normal, Anyway?

WHEN YOU HEAR THE WORD *normal*, what do you think? Does it conjure up images of a person who is able to hold down a job, who has a family and friends, and who enjoys things like going to the movies, playing sports, cooking, or any number of other hobbies? To many, a *normal* person is one who does not stray from the mainstream too much. They dress more or less like everyone else, like what other people like, and behave relatively similar to the people who surround them. A *normal* person doesn't have an unusual hairstyle or speak in a strange way or pursue interests that seem to be theirs alone. A *normal* person doesn't stray too far from widely accepted standards.

Indeed, all of those things could be considered *normal*. To wear popular fashions, to go to work five days a week, and to try to have some fun during our free time—these are all pursuits that fall within what is generally seen as the mainstream of society, that wide swath of humanity where most people dwell. To be outside of this track—to be different, to be eccentric, or to think or behave in discordant ways—is to be *abnormal*, to be less than, or to be, in some shape or form, just not good.

At least this is what we have been taught to believe. Whether it's the media or our families or simply society itself, we are reared and raised to see people who do not conform to the generally accepted rules of society as outcasts, outsiders who are often deserving of derision. Or, worse, we don't see them at all: we pretend that they don't even exist.

Think about that homeless man who stands on the corner every day, the one who's always talking to someone who isn't there. How many people walk right by him each day without a glance? Think of that kid you knew in grade school who couldn't seem to sit still at his desk for even half a class, and how the teacher told everyone else to ignore his behavior. Think about your sister, who is struck with such overwhelming sadness that she can't get out of bed for days at a time—and when she does, not one person mentions her absence.

The point is that for as many people as there are on this planet, there are an equal number of ways that people experience the world. Everyone's viewpoints, opinions, and habits are different; everyone has variations that make their existence unique from all the others.

And here's another thought for you: not everyone subscribes to the same idea of *normal*. For you it may be normal to wake up at seven o'clock every morning, take a shower, sit in rush-hour traffic, do your job for eight hours, and then go home and relax by watching TV or reading a book. For you, it's likely normal to present yourself as a clean person, as someone who bathes on a regular basis. For you, chances are it is normal to entertain mostly optimistic thoughts, to look forward to the future.

However, not everyone functions in the same capacity. For many people—for example, the 42.5 million Americans who suffer from mental illnesses[1]—a normal day is one in which they don't leave their homes because being in public brings on crippling panic attacks. Or one in which they don't shower—again—because debilitating depressive episodes have left them unable to tend to their own self-care needs. Still others find it normal not to go to work every day; in fact, they can't because of the ever-present symptoms of their mental illnesses, such as flashbacks or extreme anxiety. When you're living with mental illness, your version of normal can be quite different from what most people experience. But that does not make it any less real or valid.

---

1   Bekiempis, Victoria. "Nearly 1 in 5 Americans suffers from mental illness each year." *Newsweek* (February 28, 2014). Retrieved from http://www. newsweek .com/nearly-1-5-americans-suffer-from-mental-illness-each-year-230608 (2014).

Knowing the Difference

Having written all that, we can find some value in being able to compare the traits of a person with a mental illness to those of a person who is neurotypical, or someone who does not have any condition considered to be a mental illness. Why? Because it is in those differences that we can detect whether someone *is* suffering from a mental illness or is simply quirky or eccentric. For instance, it is neurotypical—or, if you'd rather, *normal*—to speak aloud to oneself from time to time, particularly while working out some sort of problem in one's head. Vocalizing our thoughts helps us to sort them out and helps us arrive at a conclusion to some perceived issue.

What is not *normal*—what could be a sign that the person in question has a mental illness—is appearing to be in prolonged conversation with a partner who is not there. This could be a sign that the person is having either auditory or visual hallucinations, or perhaps both. We'll define the term *hallucination* in more detail in Chapter 6, when we delve into a detailed discussion about schizophrenia and other so-called psychotic disorders. But such features are not considered normal. While being able to tolerate everyday aches and pains is a normal part of life, it's not *normal* to want to cause physical harm to one's own body. Having a good sense of, and interest in, self-preservation is healthy. Being paranoid to the point that you believe people are always watching you or are out to harm you is not.

Distinguishing between what is normal and what might be considered mental illness is fraught with fuzziness and ambiguity. Defining mental health disorders is not always a clear-cut business. We've all been sad before, so how do experts distinguish sadness from a diagnosable condition such as clinical depression? Even within the spectrum of mental health disorders, a range in severity exists. Mild depression may involve a change in appetite and a general lack of interest in regular activities, while extreme depression may involve suicidal thoughts and an inability to get out of bed. These aspects related to mental illness naturally cause confusion at times, but seeking the help of a professional who can sort them out can alleviate these frustrations and provide clarity.

Mental health disorders must be therefore distinguished from normal behaviors and categorized according to their severity. However, the circumstances surrounding any mental symptoms also must be considered in making these evaluations. It is important to appreciate that distinguishing between a normal response and a mental health disorder cannot be fully determined without knowing the person's situation. For example, grieving for weeks after the death of a loved one is perfectly normal, but having the same reaction for months without a specific trigger is not. Thus, assessing whether or not a behavior is normal also depends on the context in which it is happening.

As we wrote in the introduction, there is often a fine line between someone who is a little bit *different* and someone who has a legitimate mental illness. Is Uncle Bob just set in his ways, a creature of routine, or does his habitual checking and rechecking that the door is locked point to something more along the lines of obsessive-compulsive disorder? Is your teenage niece a picky eater, or do her frequent refusals of food mean she has some sort of eating disorder? Is your mother simply forgetful because she's getting up there in years, or does the fact that she sometimes can't remember your name mean she's in the early stages of dementia?

If you've ever asked yourself questions like these about one of your own loved ones, then you know how torturous it can be to try to tease out a diagnosis from what might be just a set of unusual personality traits. This is not to say that anyone who swerves outside the mainstream of society in any way should be evaluated for mental illness; it simply means that sometimes when the symptoms are there, we must see them for what they are and not keep excusing them or finding reasons to brush them aside. Sometimes, what seems like a mental illness really is just that. And that's okay. In fact, it's a good thing. Because once you can determine an issue is present, you're one step closer to getting your loved one the help that they will need to live as full and productive—and *normal*—a life as possible.

The Only Thing to Fear . . .

. . . is fear itself. Ever heard that one? It's an old saying and a good one, a sort of rallying cry to incite the feeling that we can overcome anything we put our minds to—that there is nothing in this world that can hold us back from achieving what we set out to do.

For those whose mental health is compromised, fear can be an ever-present factor, something to battle against on a daily basis. And it comes at the person from so many angles. There is fear of the illness itself: of its symptoms and of its getting worse in the future. There is fear of treatment: How will the medication affect me? Will I really have to tell the counselor all my deep, dark secrets? There is fear of disclosure: so many people with mental illnesses never tell anyone what they're going through because they don't know what sort of repercussions it might bring. And there's the ever-present fear of rejection: Will my family still love me if they know? Will my friends still want to be around me once they learn about my diagnosis?

And that doesn't even touch on the fear that is aimed *at* people with mental illnesses—the fear experienced by their loved ones, other people in their lives, and indeed even by strangers. To many, there is something scary about mental illness. Those who suffer from it are often seen as dangerous simply because they are the *other*, because they fall outside what we have been led to believe is the norm. They behave in ways we don't understand, and that can sometimes frighten us. Most people fear what they do not know, which is mental illness in a nutshell. There is a dearth of useful and truthful information on the topic among the general public; most people go by what they see on TV and in movies, very little of which is ever positive. The mentally ill person in popular media is always the crazed killer, the straitjacketed psychopath, or the lunatic locked up in a padded cell. He is never the friendly neighbor, the caring parent, or the loyal friend. It's no wonder people are scared.

Of course, none of this fear is founded. Yes, some mental illnesses do manifest in violence; for example, see our discussion in Chapter 6 of what drives people to commit atrocities like mass shootings. But those instances are in the minority. For every depressed pilot who commits suicide by flying a jet full of passengers into a mountain, there are millions of people with depression (or bipolar disorder, or schizophrenia, or ADHD . . .) just living their day-to-day lives and doing the best they can to keep going given what they have to work with. People with mental illnesses hold down jobs, have families, and are productive members of society. They feel happiness and pain. They love and are loved. They are, at the end of the day, just like everyone else. Most of all, they are certainly not something to be feared.

The Mental Illness Stigma

People who have mental illnesses face more challenges in life than those who do not. First and foremost, they struggle with illness itself—with symptoms and, sometimes, with side effects from the treatments they must endure. On top of that, they must deal with the stereotypes and misconceptions so many people have about individuals with mental illnesses. For example, some people believe that those with mental illnesses are somehow less intelligent, that their behaviors exist purely for attention, and that if their treatment is not "curing" them, they simply are not trying hard enough. Although most people (57 percent of those surveyed by the Behavioral Risk Factor Surveillance System[2]) feel that there is general sympathy extended toward individuals with mental illnesses, those on the receiving end report that they are not feeling that much love. Negative perceptions of people with mental illnesses are rampant in our society, leading to widespread prejudice and discrimination in the areas of employment, housing, and even health care.

All of this comprises what is known as the stigma of mental illness. *Stigma* is a label placed upon people to set them apart, to make them feel ashamed, disgraced, or embarrassed about who they are, often because of factors that are beyond their control. Those experiencing stigma are generally blamed for their own situations and made to feel

2   Centers for Disease Control and Prevention (CDC). "Attitudes toward mental illness-35 states, District of Columbia, and Puerto Rico, 2007." MMWR. Morbidity and mortality weekly report 59, no. 20 (2010): 619–625.

that they can control it or could have prevented it if only they tried a little harder. This often leads to feelings of hopelessness and distress in the stigmatized person, who, through sheer redundancy, can come to believe that others' negative views are accurate and correct. This is the awful, evil trap in which individuals with mental illnesses must operate—a cycle that works to keep them down despite their best efforts and intentions to try to live productive lives.

To what can we attribute this negativity? Where does all this misunderstanding about mental illness come from? Popular media don't help. Research has shown that on TV alone, 63 percent of references to mental health are unsympathetic, using terms such as *basket case, loony tunes, psycho,* and *crackpot* to describe people with mental illnesses.[3] Individuals with mental illnesses are often robbed of their own agency in the media, portrayed as either violent or tragic, but either way unable to control their emotions and actions. If we believe everything we see, people with mental illnesses are unpredictable, evil, foolish, incapable of rehabilitation, and, most important, absolutely unworthy of being trusted.

Given all this, is it any wonder that people with mental illnesses are sometimes resistant to confiding in others about what they experience? Understandably, because of these stigmas, they often do not make their situations known by sharing how they feel with family members or taking steps toward receiving treatment. When compared to other health conditions, mental illness ranks among the highest in terms of sufferers experiencing social stigma. However, they are not the only sufferers. We all know that individuals with HIV infections certainly experience social stigma. Similarly, lung cancer patients are commonly judged for their presumed participation in tobacco smoking, whether they smoked or not. Asthmatic children may be socially labeled as weak, unathletic, and sickly because of their respiratory limitations.

---

3   Ramsey, Mel. "There's a problem with how mental illness is portrayed on TV." *LAD Bible.com*, December 2nd, 2016. Retrieved from http://www.ladbible.com /mental-health/film-and-tv-theres-a-problem-with-how-mental-illness-is -portrayed-on-tv-20161202.

But of all these conditions, individuals with mental illness arguably suffer the highest degree of social stigma. This may be because the science related to neurologic and psychiatric illnesses is less extensive and precise when compared to other areas of medicine. In this case, ignorance is certainly not bliss for those suffering from such disorders.

The Language of Mental Illness

"Could you stop that? It's driving me crazy!"

"I am totally OCD about cleaning my house."

"I couldn't make up my mind—I was being really schizophrenic."

How many times have you made these statements or expressed these sentiments or something like them? The language of mental illness, for better or for worse, has become an everyday part of the Western language lexicon. We're constantly referring to situations as *crazy* and people as *nuts* or *bonkers* or *mental*—all of which are pejorative terms referring to mental illness. It could be argued that they're not so bad, or that they're really not referring to mental health at all—that they're simply describing someone or something that's a little bit out of the ordinary.

We all say things we don't mean literally. We use figures of speech or slang that has become engrained in our casual language, and we do so without giving it too much extra thought.

But that's probably because these words don't pertain to us. Those of us who do not suffer from mental illnesses do not and will not ever know what it's like to feel that stigma, to feel the shame, embarrassment, and isolation when someone calls another person "crazy" and laughs about it. To the person with the mental illness, there is likely not a lot of humor in their situation, and to see it treated as a joke can be extremely hurtful. Now imagine if that person is someone in your family or someone you consider a friend. That person loves you; they trust you. Hearing you say something that hurtful so flippantly could undoubtedly drive an irrevocable wedge between you and affect your relationship—and indeed the other person's life—in the most negative of ways. It's been said that language reflects beliefs, and if what that person hears is that you think being "crazy" is humorous, what are they supposed to think you really believe deep down? By discounting the word, you discount the person as well, whether you intend to or not. In this case, intention does not matter. It is the impact that counts.

The point here is to begin a thoughtful discussion about how we relate to those with mental illness, including the words that we use in everyday language. Instead of our focusing on the negative, it is more productive to take a people-first approach to language and ensure that we are valuing and affirming all people in our lives and in our communities, whether they are officially diagnosed with mental illnesses or not. For example, instead of saying a person "is OCD," we can call them an individual who has obsessive-compulsive disorder. Instead of calling someone a schizophrenic, we can refer to them as a person with schizophrenia. This might seem like a small point, but by putting the person before the illness, we change the entire focus of what we say; we're telling that person that we value them more than this one personality trait, and that we think of them as a human being before we delve into whatever mental health issues they might have. To someone who is likely used to being devalued by society as a whole, this small change can have an enormous impact. It can be the difference between someone's seeking help and remaining invisible, ashamed, and isolated from those they ought to trust the most.

Medical-Behavioral Integration

Newsflash: the head is connected to the rest of the body. While we know that's pretty obvious, we're trying to make an important point. We have to think about mental illness in the context of physical illness. Mental health issues affect physical conditions, and physical conditions can affect mental health. Medical conditions can often present with mental health symptoms: for example, hypothyroidism, which is a condition that occurs when the thyroid doesn't produce as much hormone as it should. Hypothyroidism can lead to weight gain, sluggishness, fatigue, and a low mood. This sounds a lot like major depression (to be discussed in a later chapter). If one treats hypothyroidism, the mood symptoms go away.

Whole-person health takes both mental and physical issues into account. There is much evidence that people with depression who are recovering from a heart attack have better physical health outcomes if the depression is adequately treated. While this book focuses on mental health issues, it is important to know that mental and physical health go hand in hand and cannot be separated from each other.

Chapter 2
The Epidemiology of Mental Illness

MENTAL ILLNESS IS CHALLENGING FOR the person who has it, as well as for their friends and family, but how common is this type of condition? If it were that common, surely greater awareness and attention would be present in the media and the public. Unfortunately, this does not necessarily hold true. In both of our experiences, we have seen sizable populations affected by mental health disorders, and at the same time, we have recognized shortcomings in the attention, care, and support these individuals receive. As a result, the patients we typically see in our clinics are more advanced in their illnesses than they would have been if early recognition and treatment had been employed. Many others never receive or even seek help at all.

Mental health disorders are extremely common, both in developed nations like the United States and in other countries throughout the world. Did you know that the World Health Organization (WHO) has recognized that more people in countries like the United States are disabled from mental illness than they are from heart disease or cancer? Throughout a person's lifetime, there is a 50 percent chance of developing some type of mental illness.[1] These are staggering statistics that

---

1   Reeves, William C., Tara W. Strine, Laura A. Pratt, William Thompson, Indu Ahluwalia, Satvinder S. Dhingra, Lela R. McKnight-Eily, et al. "Mental illness surveillance among adults in the United States." *MMWR Surveill Summ* 60, no. Suppl 3 (2011): 1–29.

not only show the frequency with which mental health disorders affect people and their loved ones, but also highlight the association between mental illness and disability.

Let's narrow these statistics down so they provide perspective a little closer to home. According to the National Institute of Mental Health (NIMH), the chance of any adult having a mental illness at a given point in time is roughly 18.6 percent. But before we can completely rely on this figure, we must understand that this statistic does not include mental health problems like drug abuse, alcoholism, or growth and development issues like intellectual delay or autism. In the United States alone, substance abuse and addiction affect significant numbers of people. And most of us are aware of the rise in autism over the last few decades. Regardless, taking the NIMH figures at face value, nearly one in five people has mental illness at this moment in the nation. Within this group, roughly one quarter suffer from what would be considered severe mental health conditions.[2]

Mental illness does not skip any particular group of people. However, some groups are more vulnerable than others. As a whole, mental illness appears to affect women more than men by a small margin. This may reflect the fact that fewer men seek medical help for any type of health disorder (especially mental health conditions), and therefore, women may be overrepresented in these statistics. In terms of ethnicity, Native Americans have the highest rate of mental illness at 28.3 percent, while Asian Americans have the lowest at 13.9 percent. Other ethnicities fall within these ranges. Mental illness affects all ages, including children.[3] Developed countries are not the only nations affected. According to WHO, 450 million people suffer from mental health disorders, and by 2030, depression will be the second-highest health problem in terms of costs for middle-income countries and

---

2   National Institute of Mental Health (NIMH). "Statistics." *NIMH website,* 2018. Retrieved from http://www.nimh.nih.gov/health/statistics/index.shtml.
3   Ibid.

the third highest for low-income countries.[4] Based on these statistics, the pervasiveness of mental illness within the US and throughout the world is easily appreciated.

Having established the large number of people affected by mental health problems, we can look at a few other facts and figures to further highlight their significance. For example, consider the economic cost of mental illness. Did you know that in the US alone, mental illness costs more than $300 billion annually? Direct costs related to mental illness include more than $100 billion in health-care expenses, while another $217 billion can be attributed to lost wages and disability supports. On average, each American contributes more than $1,600 per year to address the mental health problem in this country.[5] If the number of people affected by mental illness isn't enough to grab your attention, then certainly the financial costs should be.

Disability associated with mental illness is an interesting subject. From an epidemiological standpoint, disability is typically measured in "disability adjusted life years," or DALYs. This measurement refers to the total number of years lost due to a disabling illness. When mental illness is ranked alongside other major health conditions, its disability ranking is incredibly high. Mental and behavioral disorders combined account for an average of 13.6 DALYs lost. When combined with neurological disorders, this figure rises to 18.7 DALYs. For comparison purposes, heart and blood vessel disorders together average 16.8 DALYs, while cancers of all types average 15.1 DALYs.[6] This provides a clear perspective on the degree of disability individuals with mental illness experience.

4   May, Kate Torgovnick. "Some stats on the devastating impact of mental illness worldwide, followed by some reasons for hope." *TED.com blog*, September 11, 2012. http://blog.ted.com/some-stats-on-the-devastating-impact-of-mental-illness-worldwide-followed-by-some-reasons-for-hope/.

5   Substance Abuse and Mental Health Services Administration. "Projections of national expenditures for treatment of mental and substance use disorders, 2010–2020." HHS Publication No. SMA-14-4883. Rockville, MD: Substance Abuse and Mental Health Services Administration, 2014. Retrieved from https://store.samhsa.gov/system/files/sma14-4883.pdf.

6   NIMH, 2018.

Like many other health disorders, mental illness contributes to the worsening of other conditions. For example, the presence of a mental health problem is known to worsen several other chronic health disorders. Heart disease, diabetes, obesity, asthma, epilepsy, and cancer treatments are all less effective in the presence of mental illness. Just imagine a severely depressed patient with cancer struggling to go through chemotherapy. Such efforts are difficult for anyone, but even more so for someone with mental illness. Also, the rates of serious injury are between two and six times higher for individuals with mental illness compared to those without. Rates of tobacco use, alcohol abuse, and illicit drug problems similarly increase in the presence of mental illness.[7] The worsening of these other conditions in the presence of mental illness, and the indirect costs associated with mental health disorders, are not easily captured in the previously mentioned epidemiological figures. These costs are significant and should be appreciated.

Perhaps the most concerning statistic regarding mental health problems relates to suicide. Those with mental illness have much higher suicide rates, and suicide is often considered a mental health disorder in its own right. Given this, recent statistics show that the rate of suicide in the US exceeds eleven for every 100,000 people. This is so significant that suicide represents the tenth leading cause of death among all ages. Among those between eighteen and sixty-five years old, suicide is the fourth leading cause of death! In other words, suicide as a cause of death ranks higher than diabetes, stroke, homicide, and HIV infections.[8] From every epidemiological perspective, mental illness represents a serious and devastating group of health disorders.

---

7   Jané-Llopis, Eva, and Irina Matytsina. "Mental health and alcohol, drugs and tobacco: a review of the comorbidity between mental disorders and the use of alcohol, tobacco and illicit drugs." Drug and alcohol review 25, no. 6 (2006): 515–536.

8   NIMH, 2018.

Impacts of Mental Illness—Family, Community, and Society

Certainly the financial costs already mentioned affect not only those with mental illness, but also their families and society as a whole. But these statistics give an incomplete picture when considering the larger social effects mental illness can cause. From the standpoint of family members and caregivers, the burden of assisting with the care of those with mental health disorders can be significant. In order to gain a better appreciation of this, consider the following situation involving Lisa and her family:

> At twenty-four years of age, Lisa had been perfectly healthy. Working as a waitress at a busy breakfast diner, she managed to support her two young daughters and had just signed a thirty-year mortgage on a new home. But during the next few months, Lisa began making bizarre comments and acting strangely. Her conversations would often digress into the topics of aliens and God's wrath, and her associations did not always make much sense. Lisa then began neglecting her own hygiene as well as forgetting some of her daughters' appointments. At this point, Lisa's mother became concerned and stepped in to help.
>
> During the next few months, Lisa's mom had to take off work on several occasions to assist with Lisa's daughters' care. Lisa, who missed several of her shifts at the diner, was soon fired. Without the same level of income, Lisa was forced to borrow money from her sister to help pay her mortgage and other bills. Because of embarrassment at Lisa's behaviors, her longtime boyfriend, who had been living with her, decided to move out. Within the period of a few short months, Lisa's life had deteriorated significantly, and the burdens experienced by her mother, sister, and children were substantial, as well.

Lisa's story is unfortunately not an uncommon one. Family members are often called upon to fill in the gaps when mental illness affects someone. Assistance with transportation, financial support, household chores, and medical treatments requires time and energy in addition to other valuable resources. As a result, caregivers and family members are unable to pursue their own careers or jobs to the extent they normally could. A drop in income and socioeconomic status (a phenomenon known as "downward drift") often accompanies those who have a mental illness because of work problems that arise as a result of the condition. This may be further compounded, as family members may have to take off work to fill in the gap for their loved one who may be ill. Mental illness affects many others besides those with a disorder.

Because of these challenges, families with one or more individuals who suffer from mental illness naturally have a higher risk of financial struggles. Medical and health-care expenses are direct effects that increase the risk of poverty, but other indirect effects are also involved. Naturally, such situations are stressful to family members, and these factors add to the stress of managing a mental health disorder itself. As stress levels rise, family conflicts and relationship challenges also become more common, resulting in emotional and financial stress for all involved while also reducing the social support available for both the individual and their family.

Mental health problems can tear away at the fabric binding families together, and mental illness can likewise have profound effects on children of parents who suffer from such disorders. For example, a mother with postpartum depression will have a significant impact on the emotional development of her young child.[9] In some situations, mental illness may undermine good parenting and contribute to developmental disorders as well as behavioral problems within the child. If this occurs, these then add additional stresses to the home environment.

Lisa's daughters were four and six years of age at the time of her initial problems, with one in kindergarten and the

---

9   Righetti-Veltema, Marion, Elisabeth Conne-Perréard, Arnaud Bousquet, and Juan Manzano. "Postpartum depression and mother–infant relationship at 3 months old." *Journal of Affective Disorders* 70, no. 3 (2002): 291–306.

other in daycare. Though Lisa was unmarried, she had lived with her boyfriend since shortly before the birth of their first daughter, and this offered a stable home environment for both her children. But after Lisa began developing mental health symptoms and secondary effects occurred, both her daughters began showing changes in their behavior. Lisa's older daughter retreated to her room more often and was notably more quiet. A few weeks later, she began wetting the bed at night. Even her teacher noticed she was less engaged at school. Lisa's younger daughter also showed changes, with tantrums at daycare. Behavioral outbursts became so frequent, the center urged an evaluation by a pediatrician. Not only had Lisa's condition and life problems contributed to her children's behavioral changes, but she was now less well equipped to deal with such problems as a parent. Such a vicious cycle is not uncommon for many with mental health disorders.

Whether or not mental illness triggers higher stress levels for families directly or indirectly, it can lead to a vicious cycle that places these families at greater risk for ongoing difficulties. In particular, mental health disorders such as maternal depression have been linked to a variety of emotional, intellectual, and behavioral difficulties in children of people suffering from these conditions.[10] Behavior problems may be obviously disruptive, as with Lisa's younger daughter throwing tantrums at daycare, or subtler, as with Lisa's older daughter becoming more isolated, quieter, and withdrawn.

Social effects resulting from mental illness are not limited to the immediate family. Mental illness affects communities and society at large in significant ways, as well. The economic impact to society has been noted, but other secondary problems similarly cost society dearly.

---

10 Barker, Edward D., William Copeland, Barbara Maughan, Sara R. Jaffee, and Rudolf Uher. "Relative impact of maternal depression and associated risk factors on offspring psychopathology." The British Journal of Psychiatry 200, no. 2 (2012): 124–129.

More than half of all county, state, and federal prison and jail inmates suffer from some type of mental illness. According to the Bureau of Justice Statistics, not only were mental health disorders common, but less than one-third of those identified as having mental health conditions received any type of treatment before being arrested. And of these individuals, approximately three quarters met criteria for drug or alcohol abuse.[11] These impacts on society in general, and the judicial system specifically, are substantial because of the financial burden and resources required to address these problems. Imagine if treatment were provided to people with mental illness before they committed a crime. The benefits would undoubtedly be tremendous.

Perhaps one of the most significant social problems related to mental illness is homelessness. In the US, more than 3.5 million people are homeless, and one-third of these are children. In surveys conducted by the National Coalition for the Homeless, mental illness was listed as the third-most frequent cause of homelessness by most major cities. Other estimates have found that between 20 and 25 percent of all homeless people suffer from a severe mental health disorder.[12] Imagine the percentage if milder forms of mental illness were considered in these assessments! Unfortunately, mental illness may make it challenging for people to provide adequate self-care, manage a household effectively, maintain stable relationships, and keep steady work. As a result, these challenges create a higher risk for homelessness, placing yet another burden on society.

Ray's future had looked quite promising. In addition to being only one year away from a college degree in business administration, he was engaged to be married the next summer. Everything had seemed to be falling into place. But over several

---

11 Bureau of Justice Statistics. "Mental health problems of prison and jail inmates." BJS website. 2006. Retrieved from http://www.bjs.gov/content/pub/pdf/mhppji.pdf.
12 National Coalition for the Homeless. "Mental illness and homelessness." NCH website, 2009. Retrieved from http://www.nationalhomeless.org/factsheets/Mental _Illness.pdf.

months, Ray began having paranoid feelings and unusual thoughts. Soon, he was seeing and hearing things that were not real. Eventually, Ray was diagnosed with schizophrenia and underwent a variety of treatments to help his condition. Unfortunately, between his medication's side effects and his mental health symptoms, Ray often missed his daily doses and his doctor appointments. He struggled in his classes, and his relationships became increasingly strained. Within two years, Ray had dropped out of college, lost his fiancée, and continued to suffer from his mental health disorder.

Ray subsequently tried to get a job to help pay for his living expenses and his college loans, which would soon be due. After many interviews, he eventually got a job at a fast-food restaurant, but even this was fleeting: Ray was fired for missing too many days of work. Without a job, Ray was forced to ask friends and family members for help. But as the years passed, the help became less and less. His parents passed away, he had no siblings, and past friends had fallen by the wayside. At age twenty-nine, Ray found himself homeless and living on the streets, unable to stay focused on his mental health treatments, a job, or school. Ray became another statistic because of his mental health disorder.

Mental health problems may make even the simple things in life difficult. Depending on the condition, the ability to stay focused and organized in one's daily tasks can be a struggle. And when things go awry, everything seems to collapse like a row of dominoes, as demonstrated in Ray's case. One area affected by these inabilities is mental health care. Keeping appointments, taking prescribed medications, and managing health-care insurance requirements are difficult for anyone, but for those suffering from mental health disorders, these tasks can be impossible. Thus, direct health-care costs are not the only impact mental illness has on society. The difficulty individuals with mental illness have in caring for themselves contributes to the societal costs related to mental illness. By some accounts, over one-third of mentally ill patients who have received medical attention fail to follow recommended instructions.[13]

Attending to proper mental health care is only one piece of the puzzle. According to the National Institute of Health (NIH), people with severe mental illness are four times more likely to drink alcohol heavily or use illicit drugs when compared to individuals who do not have mental illness. This same group of people is five times more likely to smoke tobacco. These behaviors undermine effective mental health treatments and lead to other health problems that increase the nation's health-care burden. In contrast, treating individuals with mental health disorders early, and ensuring they take recommended meds and treatments, reduce the risk for these other problems and thus lessen the societal impact.

Perhaps the societal impact from mental health that receives the most attention is mass shootings involving shooters with known mental illnesses. Unfortunately, the list is long and seems to grow every few months. Columbine High School, Virginia Tech University, Sandy Hook Elementary, the University of California Santa Barbara, and theaters in Aurora and Lafayette are notable mass shooting events where the shooter had known mental health problems. Even more recent shootings at the Emanuel AME church in South Carolina and the Chattanooga Naval Reserve center have been attributed to the gunmen's existing mental health disorders.[14] Such tragedies represent some of the most disturbing effects mental illness can have on society, and these events further highlight a desperate need to better recognize and treat individuals suffering from mental health conditions.

---

13 Chapman, Sarah CE, and Rob Horne. "Medication nonadherence and psychiatry." Current opinion in psychiatry 26, no. 5 (2013): 446–452.
14 Crary, David. "Mental health professionals respond carefully to string of mass killings by troubled gunmen." U.S. News and World Report, July 27, 2015. Retrieved from http://www.usnews.com/news/us/articles/2015/07/27/mental-health-experts-respond-carefully-to-mass-killings.

These statistics and figures make it clear that mental illness affects many more than those who suffer from it. Family members, caregivers, friends, communities, and societies all endure primary as well as secondary effects of mental illness. Perhaps you are reading this book because you have experienced some of these effects. If so, then you are certainly not alone. Collectively, as a community, we can become better at preventing, treating, and supporting people with mental health problems and, at the same time, make positive gains to help people in their daily lives and care. The negative effects of letting mental health conditions go unattended are profound; by giving mental health disorders the same consideration as other health disorders, we as a community can make great strides in making lives and society better.

Diagnosing Mental Health Disorders—The DSM-5

If you were complaining of a persistent cough, fever, and chest pain, you would likely see your physician, who would perform an examination. In addition, perhaps hearing some abnormal breathing patterns during your chest exam, your physician might order chest X-rays, blood counts, and oxygen levels to narrow down the possible diagnoses. Based on your results, your physician would determine whether you had pneumonia, bronchitis, or some other condition accounting for your symptoms. This is the type of process we are accustomed to when it comes to medical diagnosis.

Unfortunately, such "objective" test results are not always available when it comes to mental health disorders. Many symptoms and complaints in psychiatry do not have clear findings from physical examinations, and more often than not, blood tests, head scans, and other diagnostic studies have perfectly normal results. But despite this, a person's history and their family's account can clearly indicate something is wrong with their mental functioning. So how can a psychiatrist accurately classify a mental health disorder when tangible results are lacking? This is where the *Diagnostic and Statistical Manual of Mental Disorders* (DSM) comes into play.

The DSM-1 was developed in 1952 by the American Psychiatric Association out of a need for some type of standardized format by which to classify various mental health disorders. With subsequent revisions, these manuals have increasingly developed not only common terminologies but also diagnostic criteria that must be met to secure a specific psychiatric diagnosis. The latest version is the DSM-5, which was released in 2013 and contains 157 specific mental health disorders classified within eighteen different mental health categories. It is through the use of the DSM-5 that psychiatric evaluations and diagnoses are made.

Throughout this book, we will discuss various mental health disorders in relation to the DSM-5 criteria, because these criteria have been developed based on professional observations and psychiatric research. But it is also important to note that these criteria will certainly evolve and change as science reveals more about the specific causes and changes that account for various psychiatric conditions. In the absence of more definitive lab tests and other studies, the DSM-5 currently offers the best tool to diagnose mental health disorders and to guide optimal treatments, which is why we will use this tool in describing the various mental health conditions listed in this book.

Mental Versus Medical

Though mental illnesses are clearly health disorders, inherent differences exist between physical and mental health problems that cause many to view mental health issues as less significant. For example, physical illnesses often have symptoms and findings that are more tangible when compared to mental illnesses. Someone presenting with bronchitis may likely have an abnormal lung examination, and someone with a stroke may have obvious signs of paralysis, speech dysfunction, or other obvious deficits. Likewise, many physical illnesses can be identified with abnormal test results, again making the diagnosis clearer. Unfortunately, mental illness can be more challenging in this regard. Few diagnostic lab tests, radiology studies, or other exams show abnormalities with mental health conditions. Even those that do often still fail to confirm a diagnosis. When clear-cut findings are absent, frustrations and doubts can arise. In some instances, individuals may even be suspected of faking their complaints.

Overall, people tend to be more assertive in seeking care for physical ailments than they are for mental health disorders. Many people even seek medical care when they have a persistent cold. So why wouldn't someone seek care when their thinking, mood, or behavior begins to go awry? Surveys show that the average time between the onset of mental health symptoms and the decision to seek care for those with psychotic features (hallucinations, delusions, and/or bizarre thoughts) was more than one year. For depression and anxiety symptoms, the average length of time to seek care was more than eight years![15] Making a difference in the lives of people suffering from mental illness becomes quite difficult when such a delay exists between symptoms and interventions.

We as a society tend to minimize mental health symptoms as a general rule. When compared to other conditions such as asthma or diabetes, thought or behavioral problems may be less appreciated or perhaps even ignored. After all, individuals do not necessarily want to admit something may be wrong with their thinking, mood, or behavior, particularly given the stigma associated with mental illness. Family members and friends similarly hope such problems will simply resolve on their own. Few are rushing to get the medical care needed for mental illness.

Consider the following scenario: A good friend has been down in the dumps for weeks. Nothing specifically happened to cause the blues, but regardless, he remains sullen, flat, and lethargic. Repeated attempts to get him to go cycling, out for dinner, or to a movie are met with resistance, and each time the answer is no. For many, the remedy is simply for him to "get over it." After all, it's not like he's dying of cancer or nursing a raging pneumonia. The problem seems to be simply one of willpower.

---

15 Thornicroft, Graham, Diana Rose, and Aliya Kassam. "Discrimination in health care against people with mental illness." *International Review of Psychiatry* 19, no. 2 (2007): 113–122.

Because mental illness lacks the same tangible evidence of poor health as physical ailments, often people are encouraged to simply "buck up" and get on with their lives. This is a big part of the problem. We wouldn't tell someone with a broken leg to jog it off, and we similarly shouldn't tell someone with mental health symptoms to will their symptoms away. Neither situation responds to such advice. In addition, particularly for many men, mental illness itself is seen as an inherent character weakness. People who see a "shrink" are viewed as lacking mental strength, and this undermines feelings of masculinity and pride. Unfortunately, by minimizing their complaints and trying to explain them away, these individuals delay the help they need, often causing them to become even sicker.

Mental health care can also be neglected because of how individuals and families react to mental health symptoms. Some attempt to normalize them. Individuals and families often share a form of denial in which obvious problems are shrugged off as being variants of normal. One may hear something like, "Oh, that's just Rick being Rick." In addition, some families have mental health conditions spanning several generations. When this occurs, the capacity for these families to tolerate odd thoughts and behaviors and to see them as normal increases. These are notable barriers that need to be overcome in order to encourage earlier and more comprehensive mental health care.

Because of the features of mental illness, assigning disability to someone suffering from a mental health disorder becomes challenging, as well. A doctor may hesitate in stating someone with a long-standing mental illness is disabled from working because of a lack of hard evidence in the form of exam findings and/or test results. Whether the threat is real or not, some doctors fear they may be reprimanded (or even have their licenses revoked) if some authority considers their disability assessment to be false. For these reasons, even the simple act of writing a work excuse for worsening mental health symptoms can be hard to get. All of this only serves to make the person with mental illness feel unimportant, poorly trusted, and unsupported.

Just as the medical community struggles with giving mental illness the same weight as physical illness, so does society. Employers readily excuse employees when they suffer a flu-like illness or need surgery, but calling in sick for the worsening of a depressed mood would likely be received quite poorly. Complaining that one cannot leave one's home because of an increase in obsessive-compulsive disorder (OCD) symptoms might result in being terminated. In either case, a no-win situation exists for the person with mental illness. They can either suffer through the workday in a worsened condition or face an increased risk for losing their job. Not the best situation to be in.

But all hope is not lost. Mental illness is real, and early interventions do result in better outcomes. As a result, perseverance in seeking adequate help is essential, and people with mental illness need support from their families, caregivers, friends, and communities in overcoming the natural barriers to receiving proper care that currently exist. As we learn more about psychiatric disorders, these barriers will gradually diminish. In the meantime, understanding and support are needed to help individuals suffering from mental illness to get the help they need.

Chapter 3
Mental Illness in Childhood and Adolescence

In the past, we have seen how mental illness affecting adults has received greater attention than mental health conditions affecting children. But in recent decades, disorders affecting children and teenagers have become better recognized and identified. Recent studies have shown that more than half of all mental health conditions actually begin before the age of fourteen. As many as one in every five children will experience some type of mental health problem each year.[1] Given these numbers, you can appreciate our desire to educate people about mental health disorders common to children and teens. Our goal in this chapter is to highlight the most common mental health problems in this age group. While many mental health disorders can affect children as well as adults, we will talk about a few of the most common ones as a means to increase your awareness of these conditions.

Common mental illnesses in children and teenagers include ADHD, depression, substance abuse, anxiety problems, and various conduct disorders. Attention Deficit Hyperactivity Disorder (ADHD) affects nearly 7 percent of all children, and the rising rate of children with autism spectrum disorder (ASD) has been well publicized in the

---

1   Harrison, Pam. "Mental illness on the rise in America's children." *Medscape*, 2013. Retrieved from http://www.medscape.com/viewarticle/804334.

media and within health communities.[2] While the exact causes of many of these conditions are still under investigation, your ability to appreciate symptoms and risks for these disorders offers important advantages. For one, children suffering from these symptoms may receive formal evaluations sooner. We can attest that earlier treatment often results in better outcomes for both children and their families in these situations.

Attention Deficit Hyperactivity Disorder (ADHD)

ADHD is among the more common mental illnesses affecting children, and most people readily recognize the term today. Though this condition is common in pediatric psychiatry, it can be quite difficult not only for parents, but also for educators and even physicians to recognize ADHD. For example, your sleep-deprived four-year-old may certainly show signs of irritability, restlessness, and poor concentration. But is this ADHD, or does he simply need more sleep? While there is no specific diagnostic test for ADHD, specific criteria have been developed to help doctors correctly identify this disorder. By understanding these criteria more fully, you will be better equipped to know if your child needs an evaluation for ADHD.

In essence, we recognize three different types of ADHD: a Hyperactive-Impulsive type, an Inattentive type, and a Combined type, which has features of the first two types. Hyperactive-Impulsive ADHD, as you might expect, has predominantly excessive movements and impulsivity as key symptoms. Inattentive ADHD, on the other hand, demonstrates greater problems with focus, the ability to keep things organized, and tasks that require sustained thinking. Depending on the number of symptoms present and the length of time such symptoms have been present, we may consider a diagnosis of ADHD. The following story shows a common presentation of a child with ADHD that we routinely see in practice.

---

2   Ibid.

For the last year or so, seven-year-old Deke had been a handful for his parents. At home, he was a constant bundle of energy, running and climbing over any obstacle in his way, inside or outside. Getting him to stay seated for dinner was a constant challenge, and his parents often decided not to attend church services because of his restlessness. His parents had hoped he would outgrow these behaviors, but more recently, Deke's first-grade teacher let them know Deke was constantly acting out in class and interrupting the lesson. In addition, Deke was being shunned by some of the other kids because he refused to share or take turns at recess. At the prompting of Deke's teacher, his parents decided to schedule an appointment with their pediatrician for an assessment.

Based on the symptoms and behaviors Deke was experiencing, we would suspect he indeed has the Hyperactive-Impulsive or Combined type of ADHD. In making this diagnosis, your child's doctor would go through a checklist of nine items that are considered Hyperactive-Impulsive features as well as another nine-item list of symptoms more typical of the Inattentive type. If we identify six or more of these items in either category, we would make a diagnosis of ADHD according to its type. This assumes the symptoms have been present for six months or more. With these criteria, the ability to consistently diagnose and categorize ADHD in children has greatly increased. You can better assess your own child by knowing the various items on each ADHD symptom list. The following lists show the nine criteria for each specific type of ADHD. If six or more are identified from both lists, then a Combined type of ADHD is diagnosed.

Hyperactive-Impulsive ADHD

- Fidgets/squirms
- Has difficulty being seated
- Lacks patience
- Runs/climbs excessively

- Is very talkative
- Behaves as if "driven by motor"
- Blurts out comments and answers
- Interrupts frequently
- Has difficulty sharing or taking turns

Inattentive ADHD

- Ignores details often
- Has poor ability to sustain attention
- Has poor listening abilities
- Follows instructions poorly
- Has poor organizational skills
- Loses things frequently
- Is easily distracted
- Forgets daily tasks often
- Dislikes tasks with sustained thought

Knowing the criteria by which ADHD is identified is important, since roughly one in twelve children suffer from this mental health condition.[3] Boys are more commonly diagnosed with this disorder than girls. In part, this may stem from the fact that boys often have the Hyperactive-Impulsive or Combined type of ADHD, while girls more commonly have the Inattentive type, so boys' ADHD behaviors often stand out compared to those of girls.[4] Recognizing key symptoms can thus get your child the help they need sooner rather than later.

Though there is no cure for ADHD, we have both witnessed how medications and/or behavioral therapy can significantly help ADHD children in their ability to function. Control of ADHD symptoms

---

3   NIMH(b). "Attention-Deficit/Hyperactivity Disorder (ADHD): The Basics." *NIMH Website*, 2016. Retrieved from https://www.nimh.nih.gov/health/publications/attention-deficit-hyperactivity-disorder-adhd-the-basics/index.shtml.
4   Kinman, Tricia. "Gender differences in ADHD symptoms." Healthline. 2012. Retrieved from http://www.healthline.com/health/adhd/adhd-symptoms-in-girls-and-boys#1.

allows kids to perform better in school; establish better relationships with family members and peers; and avoid other secondary problems like teen pregnancy, sexually transmitted diseases, depression, or substance abuse. Therefore, doesn't it make sense to identify children with ADHD as early as possible? By knowing which symptoms to look for, you will be able to get your child help much earlier.

At present, the exact cause of ADHD remains unknown. However, studies involving identical twins indicate genetic risks are present. Children with "ADHD genes" have been shown to have thinner areas of the brain known to affect attention and concentration.[5] At the same time, we understand that environmental triggers also exist. Children exposed to lead are at risk for ADHD, as are children born to mothers who used tobacco and/or alcohol during pregnancy.[6] These environmental risks represent a minority of cases involving children with ADHD. Until more definitive causes and cures are found, having a high level of suspicion for ADHD can help you get your child the attention they need as soon as possible.

Autism Spectrum Disorder (ASD)

As with the increased frequency of diagnosis of ADHD, we have seen the diagnosis of autism (more accurately referred to as autism spectrum disorder) increase significantly over the last several years. But is this condition really that common? According to Centers for Disease Control, autism spectrum disorder (ASD) now affects one in every sixty-eight children, and boys tend to be affected four to five times more than girls.[7] As a developmental disorder, ASD often starts before the age of two and is associated with problems in communicating, interacting socially, and performing repetitious behaviors. In our experience, children with ASD have difficulty, ranging from mild to severe,

---

5 NIMH(b), 2016.
6 Ibid.
7 NIMH(c). "Autism Spectrum Disorder" *NIMH Website*, 2018. Retrieved from https://www.nimh.nih.gov/health/topics/autism-spectrum-disorders-asd/index .shtml.

in interacting and talking with other people. In the milder cases, we often see parents delay seeking help in hopes that the behavior will simply go away. This delay reduces the potential benefits of treatment, since earlier interventions have been shown to improve function.[8]

It is important for you to appreciate typical ASD symptoms, but these will vary with a child's age. The diagnosis of ASD typically requires assessments by behavioral pediatricians or by psychiatric and/or neurologic specialists, but often it may be the parent of the child, or the pediatrician, who first identifies a child as failing to attain developmental milestones. Numerous screening assessments and questionnaires now exist to help provide better accuracy and consistency in diagnosing ASD. We have seen how these tools give ASD children a better chance of getting help earlier in life. Emily provides a good example of the benefits of early intervention for ASD:

> For the last few months, Emily's parents had noticed her tendency to focus on a specific few toys in her room, but because she was only three, they thought little about it at first—what three-year-old girl doesn't like her toys? But they became more concerned when Emily started to throw tantrums when her daily routine was changed. Even the specific way her teeth were brushed became an issue. The final straw came when Emily's mom noticed that Emily would never engage with the other kids during her play dates in the neighborhood. The next week, she scheduled an appointment with the pediatrician.
>
> During the doctor's visit, Emily was confirmed to be of normal height and weight, and she had met all of her age-appropriate motor milestones. In other words, she was able to run, ride a tricycle, and climb with other kids her age. But her language skills were less developed, and her vocabulary was not as broad as it should be. During the appointment,

---

8   Ibid.

Emily failed to make eye contact with the doctor and clung to a doll she had brought with her throughout the visit. After a few additional referrals, and the completion of some screening tests, Emily was diagnosed as having mild ASD. After ongoing, regular behavioral therapy sessions, Emily was able to advance to kindergarten a couple of years later.

Though Emily's symptoms were rather vague, her parents astutely noticed that her social skills and interactions were a little off. As a result, a diagnosis was made and treatments were started, allowing improvements to occur. Knowing ASD symptoms can allow you and your child the same opportunity. Though severity varies, ASD children struggle with social abilities and tend to prefer the same routine and patterns of behavior every day. For a young child, this may involve poor eye contact, difficulty sharing toys, paying attention to objects more than people, and unusual emotional reactions. For older children, trouble interacting with peers at school, repetitive behaviors, and social isolation may be more evident. In some cases, ASD children may even regress and lose cognitive or social skills that they once had. Because of this variation, any persistent behaviors that show poor social interactions and inflexibility to change should alert you to the possibility of ASD.

Over the course of the last several years, we have seen a dramatic rise in the incidence of ASD. For example, in 2000, the CDC reported that about one in every 150 children had autism, but by 2006, this figure rose to one in every 110 children, and in 2012, one in every 88 children. Better diagnosis, greater awareness, and a broader definition of ASD account for some of this increase, though we do not know to what degree. The expansion of community, school, and private services and treatments for ASD has also helped facilitate greater recognition.[9] At

---

9   Park, Alice. "Autism rises: More children than ever have autism, but is the increase real?" *Time*, March 29, 2012. Retrieved from http://healthland .time.com/2012/03/29/autism-rises-more-u-s-children-than-ever-have-autism -is-the-increase-real/.

the same time, we believe other factors are present that have made ASD more common in children. These other factors are currently unknown, so it remains important that you and other parents have a heightened level of suspicion for ASD.

Though the cause of ASD remains unknown, studies involving identical twins with ASD show a 90 percent rate of occurrence. Likewise, brothers and sisters of children with ASD are thirty-five times more likely to develop ASD than others.[10] In our opinion, this strongly supports a genetic component to the disorder. But at the same time, triggers in the environment are suspected and are likely necessary for genes to express the mental disorder. To date, a clear environmental role (including childhood vaccinations) has *not* been identified. So for now, we continue to stress early diagnosis and intervention. Through early interventions, children with ASD have shown to have improved intellect, language skills, and a better ability to adapt to change.[11] By understanding the basics of this mental illness, and by being proactive in its evaluation, you can play a key role in achieving a better outcome for your child.

Depression in Childhood

You might think of depression as predominantly an adult mental health condition. But we have seen children, and particularly teenagers, commonly suffering from this condition, as well. Based on various studies, between 1 and 2 percent of children suffer depression before the age of puberty; this figure then rises to as high as 6 percent for adolescents.[12] Thus, it is important for you to appreciate common symptoms of childhood depression. In addition to the high number of children affected by depression, this mental illness can lead to many other mental health problems. For one, depression in children increases

---

10 Ibid.

11 Ibid.

12 Giardino, Angelo. "Pediatric depression." *Medscape*, 2014. Retrieved from http://www.medscape.com/viewarticle/804334.

the chances of depression as an adult. Suicide risks, as well as alcohol and drug abuse, also become more likely when depression is present.[13]

How is depression diagnosed in a child? Like many mental health disorders, we diagnose depression based on the presence of specific symptoms for a minimum length of time. Based on the DSM-5, the presence of five or more depression-related symptoms must be present for two continuous weeks or more to support a diagnosis of depression. Of these five symptoms, one must be either a depressed mood or a loss of interest or pleasure in activities. Likewise, symptoms must cause a significant amount of distress and/or result in difficulties performing regular daily responsibilities. For children, however, the symptoms of depression may not be as straightforward when compared to those of adults:

> Zack had just entered high school, and despite the new environment, his parents presumed he would adjust well. After all, Zack had always made friends without any difficulty, and he had always done well in school. But after several weeks in ninth grade, Zack began complaining of headaches and difficulty sleeping. His appetite seemed to have slipped, as had his grades. A visit to the doctor failed to reveal anything specific, but the symptoms persisted despite reassurance from the doctor. Zack's parents began to notice he would spend more and more time in his room alone, and weekends were no longer filled with movie outings with friends. Perplexed and frustrated, eventually Zack's parents insisted on another evaluation by the doctor.

Zack's case may not be typical for many children or teenagers suffering from depression, but such presentations are common nonetheless. In our clinical experiences, we often see children complain of symptoms like headaches, stomachaches, or other physical ailments when depression exists. Increased time alone, reduced time with friends, and

---

13 Ibid.

irritability can also be more common in children with depression.[14] Other depressive symptoms may also be present, but these physical complaints may attract more of your attention and reduce the chances of considering depression as a cause. Therefore, a high level of suspicion is needed when it comes to a diagnosis of depression in children.

Fortunately, we have witnessed significant advances in the treatment of depression. With the discovery that children with depression often have lower levels of some specific brain chemicals (like serotonin, dopamine, and norepinephrine), medications that boost these levels have been beneficial. By combining these treatments with various types of psychological therapy for the child, adolescent, and family, we have been further able to improve moods and levels of daily function. As new discoveries are made, such therapies continue to improve. Of course, we cannot treat what is not diagnosed. By having a greater awareness of key depression symptoms and features, you can help significantly in diagnosing and treating this common childhood condition.

DSM-5 Criteria for Depression
- Depressed mood
- Loss of interest or pleasure in activities
- Sleep disturbances (increased or decreased)
- Weight and appetite changes
- Reduced ability to concentrate
- Agitation
- Fatigue and loss of energy
- Feelings of guilt and worthlessness
- Suicidal thoughts

While depression can be significant in terms of causing distress for many children, we must make special mention of depression and the risk for suicide in this age group. We appreciate suicide as a notable risk, particularly for teens with depression. Suicide is the third-leading

---

14 Ibid.

cause of death in both children and adolescents.[15] Given that depression is a primary factor in these children, the risk of suicide demands our attention if depressive symptoms exist. As previously mentioned, depression is also associated with higher usage of alcohol, tobacco, and illicit drugs.[16] While not all cases of substance abuse reflect underlying depression, many times we see these mental health conditions coexist. Thus, treating depression will often also help in treating substance abuse problems.

Social Media and Childhood Mental Health Issues

You are likely aware that kids of all ages are actively involved in the internet and social media today. Social media use is the most common activity enjoyed by children and teenagers currently. Over 75 percent of children own a cellular phone, the majority use it to access social media daily, and nearly one quarter log in to these sites more than ten times a day![17] These are impressive numbers. Because social media and internet access are so common among children, the effects on their mental health, both good and bad, need to be considered.

Certainly, we can appreciate how many positive benefits come with children's use of social media. Social media encourage community engagement and involvement, and they boost creativity and new ideas. With such a broad reach, social media also encourage diversity while promoting independence and an awareness of one's identity. We have seen how social media and the internet have created new resources and opportunities for learning for children. Even health information, including information about mental illness, has been made more accessible.

Unfortunately, some unhealthy effects from social media can also involve children. From our perspective, one of the most concerning effects is that of cyberbullying. Cyberbullying is defined as using social

---

15 Ibid.
16 Ibid.
17 O'Keeffe, Gwenn Schurgin, and Kathleen Clarke-Pearson. "The impact of social media on children, adolescents, and families." Pediatrics 127, no. 4 (2011): 800–804.

media, or other electronic media, to share false, hostile, or embarrassing information or images regarding another person. We see this practice all too frequently. Among all the potential health risks, cyberbullying represents the most common risk to your child online. It has been linked to depression, anxiety, social isolation, and even suicide.[18] Within a short period of time, we have seen this mental health concern become remarkably common.

Cyberbullying, however, is not the only mental health concern associated with social media. Other mental health problems we see include sexting (sending, receiving, and forwarding sexually implicit messages or images), loss of privacy, internet addiction, and sleep deprivation conditions. A condition known as "Facebook depression" has even been described as resulting from the intensity, pressure, and eventual isolation stemming from the use of Facebook and other social media sites too much.[19] Each of these social media effects creates specific concerns for your child and his or her mental well-being, and recognizing such risks represents the first step you can take in addressing these potential problems.

Solutions in addressing childhood mental health conditions associated with social media require parents to actively engage with their children. You may lack the technical skills to keep up with your kids' activities online, or you simply might not have the time to devote to social media to the extent it would take to oversee your child's online behaviors. But you can be aware of the potential effects social media can have on your child's mental health. By dedicating time to having conversations about social media, establishing limits and boundaries for its use, and getting more involved in social media sites, you can better protect your child from negative consequences, and should any of the negative effects described here occur, your efforts will promote earlier recognition that professional help may be needed.

18 Ibid.
19 Ibid.

The Impact of Childhood Trauma

What children experience during childhood can have a lasting impact throughout their lifetime, and this includes both positive and traumatic experiences. Childhood is a time in which the mind and body make significant developmental gains. Research studies have shown that severe stress experienced during this period can not only have a negative impact on a child's developing brain, but also adversely affect physical health outcomes across their lifespan.

Much of this data was revealed in the Adverse Childhood Experiences Study (ACES).

This study, conducted in the mid-1990s, examined health outcomes in adults assigned to a health maintenance organization (HMO). These study participants were asked about their exposure to severe trauma during childhood, including negative experiences such as physical abuse, sexual abuse, emotional abuse, emotional neglect, parental separation, parental divorce, parental incarceration, domestic violence, and/or living with a parent who had substance abuse or mental illness. What the researchers found was both astonishing and impactful—specifically, the more of these very specific traumatic events one experienced during childhood, the more likely they were at risk for poorer health outcomes in adulthood. The risk of later heart disease, stroke, hepatitis, lung disease, depression, suicide attempt, and even premature death is greatly increased if severe trauma is experienced during childhood.

> Shirley was a bright child who loved to read, sew, and play with her eight siblings. She was active and had dreams of becoming a dancer or teacher. Her father, a hardworking and proud family man, was a stoic provider for his large family. He was also an alcoholic. Shirley has vivid memories of watching her father drink himself into an angry alcoholic rage. She would often witness, as a young child, her drunken father becoming physically abusive toward her mother or verbally taking his rage out on one of the children (including Shirley). When intoxicated,

he would become very scary and threaten them all with a loud, angry tirade. Though she has many fond memories of times with her mother and siblings, Shirley describes her childhood as filled with chaos and fear (of her father). Shirley witnessed domestic violence and alcoholism, both at the hands of her father, throughout her childhood and teen years.

Fast-forwarding to Shirley's adult life, we find that her physical health has suffered several challenges. Despite a fairly adequate diet and exercise regimen, she was diagnosed with high blood pressure in her thirties. In her early fifties, despite proper treatment of her blood pressure, Shirley suffered a debilitating stroke. In fact, she has suffered at least two strokes as an adult and has residual paralysis and limited functioning in several areas of her life.

Can we definitively say that Shirley's childhood experience of domestic violence, emotional abuse, and parental alcoholism are the causes of her significant cardiovascular disease several decades later? *No.* However, this argument can definitely be made, supported by scientific data and evidence as demonstrated in ACES.

* * *

Children are often resilient, especially if they develop a support system that includes a strong family, mentor, educational system, and/or community. Yet the research and evidence are clear. Toxic levels of stress, caused by negative childhood experiences, can derail healthy brain development and increase one's risk of later developing dozens of chronic illnesses. The bottom line: childhood adversity and trauma dramatically affect health across a lifetime.

Psychiatric Medications in Children

A conservative approach is best when considering the use of psychiatric medications as part of an integrated treatment plan for children and adolescents living with mental health conditions. There are instances in which medication therapy offers the youth relief from symptoms and significantly improves challenging behaviors. We recommend that parents and families carefully consider medication management for pediatric mental health conditions. The prescribing of psychiatric medications in this special population should always be done under the guidance of a well-trained and skilled clinician, such as a child and adolescent psychiatrist or a developmental-behavioral pediatrician.

Better Understanding, Better Awareness, and Better Mental Health

While the topics we covered in this chapter are far from comprehensive, the more common conditions involving this age group have been highlighted. Based on this information, in addition to the information outlining the negative impact of significant childhood trauma, we hope a common theme can be appreciated. For most childhood mental health problems, earlier diagnosis leads to earlier interventions, which lead to better responses to treatment. Because some of these conditions may demonstrate unusual or subtle features, understanding common symptoms and the basic criteria of these illnesses can greatly help you as a parent.

Compared to the past, greater awareness and recognition of childhood mental health disorders exist today. This is evident in the increased diagnosis as well as treatment of conditions like ADHD and ASD. While we don't believe this to be the only cause of the increased occurrence of these conditions, the benefits of earlier diagnosis are readily appreciated. However, we still have a long way to go. Many children and adolescents never see a professional for their complaints, and many may not even share their problems with their parents or others. Hopefully, the information provided in this chapter gives you a better grasp of each of these common mental health disorders, which will increase your ability to recognize possible signs and features of common childhood mental health problems.

Chapter 4
Mood Disorders

MOST PEOPLE HAVE EXPERIENCED MOOD fluctuations. Sleep deprivation, various stresses, a sore throat, and many other factors can contribute to normal ups and downs. Probably every person alive can relate to that. But how can you tell if someone's mood changes have gone beyond the normal ups and downs of life and progressed into more serious issues that require medical attention? An actual mood disorder is characterized by changes in mood with greater intensity, severity, and duration than what most people experience as they go through life. Variations in human behaviors exist, so it is sometimes difficult to tell when changes in mood go beyond the range of what is considered normal. Despite being extremely common, these disorders often go undetected and undiagnosed, which keeps people from receiving effective treatment and getting the help they need to live happy, stable, and productive lives. We want to address the more common mood disorders so those suspected of having such troubles can get the medical help they deserve. In this chapter, we will discuss major depression, bipolar disorder, and seasonal affective disorder.

Major Depression

Among all the mood disorders, major depression is one of the most common. Major depression causes the highest degree of disability among its sufferers: nearly 16 million people in the US suffer from it, nearly 7 percent of the population.[1] As psychiatrists, both of us have diagnosed and treated many people with depression, but many such people never seek or receive the care they need. Instead, they go through their daily lives struggling with the symptoms of depression, which makes even the simplest tasks difficult. But there is good news. About 80 percent of people with depression can be effectively treated with proper therapy.[2] Our goal is to educate people about major depression so those with this mental health condition can receive the treatment they need.

What causes depression? Many people falsely believe that traumatic life events (such as the death of a loved one, a divorce, or a major car accident) actually cause depression. While these events often cause people to be sad, they do not cause depression in the majority of people. In fact, despite major depression being a common mental health problem, its precise cause has yet to be well defined. However, studies have shown that genetics do play a partial role. In studying twins, researchers have found that if one has depression, then the risk of the other twin having it is about 40 to 50 percent. And if you are a first-degree relative of someone with depression, your risk is increased threefold.[3] Clearly, some degree of genetic risk is present. Despite these statistics, genetics do not entirely explain why depression occurs. Chronic pain, stress, lack of sleep, and some specific medical illnesses also trigger depression in many people. We have seen depression commonly associated with Parkinson's disease, multiple sclerosis, stroke, cancer, and even heart disease. Likewise, people who have thyroid dysfunction or memory disorders often have depression. So, while genes may make you more likely to get depression, life experiences and other conditions can also increase your risk. In other words, it's not just nature—it's nurture, too.

---

1   National Institute of Mental Health (NIMH(d)). "What is depression?" *NIMH website*, 2018. Retrieved from https://www.nimh.nih.gov/health/topics/depression/index.shtml.

2   Halverson, Jerry L. "Depression." *Medscape*, 2019. Retrieved from http://emedicine.medscape.com/article/286759-overview.

3   Ibid.

How do you know if you have major depression? For psychiatrists, making the diagnosis requires asking specific questions about a number of specific symptoms and complaints. People with major depression must have at least five or more depressive symptoms lasting a minimum of two weeks, and at least one of these symptoms must be a depressed mood or a loss of interest in normal activities the person likes to do. The other symptoms common to major depression include significant changes in weight or appetite, problems with sleeping, being overly tired, having no energy, being restless or sluggish, feeling worthless, and/or constantly thinking about death or suicide. You can see how these would be common features of depression, but unless people are specifically asked about these issues, they may never be diagnosed.

LaDawn had just turned thirty and seemed to have it all. Her interior design business had been thriving, and she deeply cared for her husband and two children. But during the last few months, LaDawn had been unable to shake a persistent feeling of unhappiness. At first, she thought she was just reacting to some financial stresses related to refinancing her home. But as the weeks passed, the feelings persisted. Her sadness became so overwhelming that she no longer wanted to participate in the weekly family trips to the farmer's market, and she had completely lost interest in cycling, which she previously had loved. In addition, she had begun to dread nighttime because she was having difficulty sleeping. She started gaining weight, which did not help her self-esteem, and she seemed to care less and less about life in general.

If it had been up to LaDawn, she might have never sought help. But her husband noted the progressive change in LaDawn's mood and behavior. Not only had she lost interest in normal life activities, but she had also let things slip at work, which had always been her passion. Her husband was also aware that LaDawn's mother had suffered depression later in life. After coaxing her repeatedly, he was eventually able to get LaDawn to have an evaluation. After being diagnosed with major depression, LaDawn was prescribed medication that significantly improved her symptoms over a period of a few weeks.

What was the exact cause of LaDawn's depression? From the story, it is a little difficult to tell. But in all likelihood, stress and genetics probably played a role. Her story highlights the role family members and friends play in helping people with depression get the care they need. If LaDawn's husband had not been so observant, she might have continued to avoid going to the doctor. We have seen how untreated depression can get worse and worse and cause people to have all kinds of life problems. Relationships are often affected, and other medical illnesses tend to respond to treatments less well. Also, self-medication with drugs and alcohol can occur. Alcohol itself is a depressant. People use alcohol to temporarily escape their "depressed world," but over time, alcohol actually makes their depression worse. Knowing the symptoms and encouraging health evaluations for people with depression are very important so these unwanted secondary problems can be avoided.

In regard to treatment, science has made great strides in discovering several medications that help with depression. You have probably heard of many of these. But what you may not know is that these medications work by adjusting specific neurochemicals in the brain. By increasing levels of serotonin, norepinephrine, and/or dopamine, these medications help eliminate depression in many people. This is because major depression has been linked to low levels of these substances. Likewise, various types of psychological therapy (talk therapy) can also be used to help with the symptoms of depression. In understanding that effective treatments exist, you can better appreciate why it is important for people with depression to be evaluated as soon as possible.

Unfortunately, some myths exist about depression. For example, you might suspect depression is always a lifelong disorder. While it certainly can be a chronic condition, major depression can occur as a single episode in life lasting only a period of weeks to months.

In fact, only half of the people with a single episode of depression will have additional episodes in the future.[4] Also, most people do not appreciate that many treatable causes of depression exist. Side effects from some medications can cause a depressed state. We have often seen how some people with bipolar disorder (discussed below) are misdiagnosed with major depression. Because of the number of medical conditions associated with depression, we encourage anyone suffering from depressive symptoms to seek medical assessment sooner rather than later. Not only does this allow effective treatment sooner, but it may also identify some other condition that needs urgent attention.

Bipolar Disorder

You have probably also heard of bipolar disorder. But while the symptoms of depression are understood by most people, those of bipolar disorder (also known as manic depression) often cause some degree of confusion. You have likely heard the term tossed around in casual conversation, but what exactly does *bipolar* mean? The best way to understand it is to think of the two extremes of someone's moods. On one "pole," a person may experience a mood that is depressed and sad; on the other "pole," their mood may be extremely happy and euphoric. In essence, these two moods reflect the two sides of bipolar disorder. While we may be making this a little too simple, this perspective helps provide a basic framework in understanding this common mood disorder.

Exactly how common is bipolar disorder? Though not as common as major depression, bipolar disorder still affects many people: nearly 4 percent of the population suffers from it, and this is probably an underestimation.[5] Unlike depression, which may occur as a single transient episode, bipolar disorder tends to be lifelong. Of those who develop

---

4 Burcusa, Stephanie L., and William G. Iacono. "Risk for recurrence in depression." *Clinical psychology review* 27, no. 8 (2007): 959–985.

5 Soreff, Stephen. "Bipolar affective disorder." *Medscape*, 2018. Retrieved from http://emedicine.medscape.com/article/286342-overview.

bipolar disorder, half have symptoms before twenty-five years of age.[6] You might think these statistics are pretty depressing themselves. However, with proper treatment, people with bipolar disorder typically lead very productive lives and do quite well. Thus, while bipolar disorder is chronic and requires ongoing attention, we can reassure you that it can be well treated in most instances.

As with major depression, the exact cause of bipolar disorder is not known. It has been found that first-degree relatives of people with bipolar disorder have a higher incidence of developing the illness. This supports genetics as a partial factor in its occurrence. Also, some studies have shown that the very front part of the brain is often smaller in bipolar disorder patients compared to those without the condition. Specific changes in the brain's structure may therefore be a reason for the mood fluctuations and other symptoms in this condition.[7] Genetics may increase the risk, but other factors (yet to be found) are also required for it to occur.

What is bipolar disorder, and what does it look like? These are the important questions. In essence, two major types of bipolar disorder exist, bipolar I and bipolar II. To understand the difference between these types, you must understand the difference between mania and depression. Depressive symptoms are the same ones we previously described when discussing major depression: feelings of sadness and hopelessness, a loss of interest in pleasurable activities, excessive fatigue and loss of energy, restlessness or sluggishness, reduced memory and concentration abilities, changes in weight and appetite, changes in sleep, and/or recurring thoughts about death or suicide. Just as in major depression, these depressive symptoms must last for a period of at least two weeks to be considered relevant in bipolar disorder.

Manic symptoms, on the other hand, can be viewed as the "polar" opposite of depressive symptoms. If you're feeling the opposite of

6   National Institute of Mental health (NIMH(e)). "Bipolar disorder?" *NIMH website*, 2016. Retrieved from https://www.nimh.nih.gov/health/topics/bipolar-disorder/index.shtml.

7   Soreff, 2015.

depressed, then you are likely feeling extremely happy. In mania, people must have changes in mood within high levels of "happiness" to the point of euphoria. Irritability is also commonly present. In addition, bipolar individuals with mania also must have at least three other associated symptoms such as a reduced need for sleep, excessive talking, an increase in pleasure-related activities, exaggerated ideas, rapid changes in thoughts, and/or an inability to stay focused. These symptoms must last at least one week. If these symptoms exist, then the manic aspect of bipolar disorder is confirmed.

You might think that everyone with bipolar disorder has manic symptoms, but this is not always the case. For example, if manic complaints (as described above) last less than a week (but at least four days), then the person is described as being "hypomanic." The presence of mania versus hypomania determines whether a person is diagnosed with Type I or Type II bipolar disorder. Accurate diagnosis can help provide information to these individuals and their families, and it can help in choosing the best treatments. But because hypomania is less obvious to some people, delayed diagnosis or even misdiagnosis can occur.

So what is the difference between the two types of bipolar disorder? It can be rather subtle. Type I bipolar disorder occurs equally in men and women. Based on our experience, this type is more easily diagnosed once people who suffer from it finally get to a doctor, because those with Type I have manic symptoms that are often easy to recognize. There is one problem: because depression may be absent in Type I, people may not seek a doctor's evaluation. They enjoy the exaggerated happiness and euphoria associated with the manic mood, and because manic symptoms can enhance productivity, reduce the need for sleep, and provide feelings of elation, they may not trigger medical assessment. But these mood symptoms are not without their problems. Often, manic phases result in many difficulties: problems related to one's job, school performance, and relationships are typical for people suffering from mania. These individuals should receive medical evaluation and treatment as soon as possible.

In contrast, Type II bipolar disorder has prominent features of depression without an obvious manic phase. Hypomanic periods of less than one week's duration occur, which may be less noticeable. Because these hypomanic phases may be minimized or ignored by individuals and their families, we often see Type II bipolar individuals misdiagnosed as having major depression. This highlights why it is important for you to encourage those you love with mood problems to seek medical evaluation. With the correct diagnosis, they can receive the right treatments. Otherwise, their mood condition persists, resulting in ongoing problems.

Tricia had begun her second year of college, and she had always excelled in her classes. But lately, she was having difficulty concentrating and staying motivated. Friends noticed she no longer participated in many of her usual activities, and Tricia herself knew she had lost interest in keeping up with her social circles. Often, she would feel dejected and sad, and this only seemed to be worsened by her ever-present insomnia. At times, it got to the point where she would even contemplate ending her life. But these episodes never lasted for extreme periods of time. After a few weeks, they would often improve, despite Tricia's knowing they would recur further down the road.

Two months into her classes that year, Tricia had a fairly sudden change in her mood. Instead of being tired and depressed, she began having an abundance of energy. She engaged in conversations with strangers, which would go on for hours. Not only did she resume many of her activities with her friends, she joined three new clubs. Despite this energy boost, her ability to concentrate got worse, as did her grades. Her friends noticed how Tricia's stories were very disconnected and often did not have a point. In addition, she would often go off on tangents about how she had received a calling from God to help unborn children. Friends soon began making excuses in order to avoid her. While Tricia had been fairly frugal in the past, suddenly she was charging clothes, jewelry, and electronics to her credit cards despite having no additional sources of income. After a week of these behaviors in Tricia, her sister noticed the dramatic changes in Tricia and insisted she go to her doctor.

Tricia clearly had depression-type symptoms initially, but after several weeks, she began having a completely different set of problems. You can likely appreciate that the increase in energy, reduced need for sleep, and excessive talking are more consistent with manic symptoms. Since these lasted more than one week, Tricia likely has Type I bipolar disorder. You may also appreciate the challenge in diagnosing bipolar disorder. Despite Tricia's manic symptoms being a marked change from her depressive ones, and despite these lasting more than one week, her friends tended to shy away from her. Tricia likewise may have been enjoying her newfound energy and elevated mood, but mania can be just as detrimental as depression in causing life problems. Fortunately, her sister insisted on Tricia's seeking the medical attention she needed.

The good news is that bipolar disorder can be treated very effectively. Through the use of mood-stabilizing medications and talk therapies, mood swings can be smoothed out and controlled. This allows people with bipolar disorder to function normally again. But we must stress the importance of ongoing treatment. For bipolar individuals who do not receive or continue treatment, several problems can occur. In addition to normal life challenges, the risk for drug and alcohol abuse is significant, and mood changes (both highs and lows) often become worse over time in the absence of medical care. For these reasons, getting the proper care sooner rather than later is critical so those with bipolar disorder can regain the ability to lead normal lives.

Seasonal Affective Disorder

Are you someone who dreads a cloudy, dreary day? Or maybe you seem to always get a little down during the winter months. For some people, these symptoms reflect a mood disorder known as seasonal affective disorder, or SAD. Seasonal affective disorder is more than simply feeling a little glum on occasion because you cannot get outdoors and enjoy warmer weather. This condition is a tendency for people with major depression, or with depressive symptoms in bipolar disorder, to develop depression during specific seasons of the year. Based on recent estimates, more than half a million people in the US alone have seasonal affective disorder, and of these, three quarters are women.[8]

Based on our experience, seasonal affective disorder most commonly starts in the fall, worsens during the winter, and then begins to subside in the spring. You might suspect that colder temperatures cause this condition, but actually, temperature has nothing to do with it. Instead, the primary factor is the amount of sunlight one is exposed to. As the amount of daily sunlight decreases, depressive mood symptoms become more common. People living at higher latitudes, where sunlight exposure is the least during winter months, have a greater risk for developing this condition.[9]

Why would sunlight, or rather a lack of it, trigger depression in some people? Our biological clocks depend on light exposure to regulate many things within our bodies. Depending on the amount and timing of sunlight (or bright light) exposure, changes in our moods, hormone levels, and sleep patterns occur. Some evidence suggests that light exposure also affects the levels of specific neurochemicals in our brains, which may explain why this disorder develops and offer new ways to treat the condition.

People with seasonal affective disorder face considerable challenges. Just like major depression, seasonal affective disorder triggers the same symptoms and difficulties. Unlike depression, the treatment for seasonal affective disorder involves providing adequate light exposure so that mood changes may resolve. This fact highlights why medical

---

8 Cleveland Clinic. "Seasonal depression." Cleveland Clinic Website, 2016. Retrieved from http://my.clevelandclinic.org/services/neurological_institute/center-for-behavorial-health/disease-conditions/hic-seasonal-depression.

9 Ibid.

assessment and accurate diagnosis is important. In our experience, the use of a 10,000-lux light box (known as light therapy) effectively treats most people with this condition when used regularly. Light therapy, combined with exercise and occasionally the use of behavioral therapy, allows people to manage their seasonal mood changes well. If you know of someone with symptoms that fit this disorder, encourage them to seek a formal evaluation as soon as possible.

Do I Have a Mood Disorder? Or Am I Just Moody?

After reading about the more common mood disorders described in this chapter, you should be better able to answer these questions. For major depression and bipolar disorder, specific symptoms and durations of complaints must exist to identify the condition. But not everyone recognizes these symptoms themselves, and some simply choose not to seek medical attention. We have often seen people suffer from mood-related problems for years before presenting for treatment or eventually ending up in an emergency room. Depression symptoms may have been minimized, ignored, or thought to be too insignificant in nature. Manic features were often not considered a problem or were not well recognized by family and friends. These are the most common obstacles such individuals face in getting the medical care they need.

Unlike the temporary changes in mood that everyone experiences, actual mood disorders interrupt the ability to carry out normal, daily responsibilities on a regular basis. This may involve one's ability to maintain stable relationships, or it may interfere with the ability to perform expected tasks at work or in school. Awareness of these problems with normal function is thus required when making the diagnosis of a mood disorder. Any mood changes that cause such functional challenges should prompt a decision to seek professional help.

If symptoms of depression last for two weeks or longer, we encourage people to arrange for an evaluation. Likewise, if manic symptoms are recognized, assessment should be sought, as well. Based on our experience with these conditions, earlier diagnosis results in better treatment both in the short term and down the road, avoiding many of the

problems that can develop later. Earlier diagnosis and treatment also
allow a better quality of life for these individuals and greater opportunities to reach their goals. With a better understanding of these mood
disorders, you have the tools necessary to recognize their presence and
seek the help needed, whether it is for yourself or your loved ones.

Chapter 5
Anxiety Disorders

EVERYONE WORRIES FROM TIME TO time. Anxiety is a normal emotion that helps us prepare for an examination, get ready for a presentation, or anticipate problems. But sometimes, anxiety and similar emotions can become exaggerated or excessive in nature, and this forms the basis for a number of anxiety disorders, including generalized anxiety disorder, various types of phobias or exaggerated fears, obsessive-compulsive disorder, panic disorder, and post-traumatic stress disorder. In this chapter, we will provide you with a better understanding of these mental health problems so you can more easily recognize them and help those around you get the care they need.

What exactly are anxiety disorders? These disorders are categorized as having a major component of increased anxiety or worry. Some anxiety conditions consist of obsessive-compulsive disorders. Others involve stress-related or trauma-related anxiety states in which some type of major stress or trauma triggers abnormal amounts of anxiety. While it is beyond the scope of this chapter to discuss all the types of anxiety disorders, we will describe the more common ones so you can better understand them. As a result, you will gain an appreciation for the causes, features, and treatment options of each of these disorders.

Generalized Anxiety Disorder

Let's start with one of the most common anxiety disorders. Generalized anxiety disorder (GAD) is a condition associated with an excessive degree of anxiety and worry affecting many areas of one's life. You might be amazed at how many people are actually affected by GAD— in the US alone, nearly seven million people have GAD at any given time, which is essentially 3 percent of the population![1] While GAD can develop at any age, it begins for most people during their teenage years or young adulthood. This anxiety disorder can therefore affect people's ability to function during some of their most highly productive years.

When a doctor is making a diagnosis of GAD, the symptoms described provide the most important clues. As you might imagine, worrying is a major component of this condition. Excessive worry or anxiety must have been present for six months or longer in order for someone to be diagnosed with GAD, and at least three other common complaints associated with this condition must be present, such as restlessness, fatigue, difficulty concentrating, irritability, muscle tightness, and/or sleep problems (particularly insomnia). People with GAD also describe many physical complaints: muscle aches, tremors, muscle twitches, headaches, dizziness, nausea, and even hot flashes. Of course, these symptoms may have other causes, and it is important to make sure that other medical problems are not present. Screening for other causes of a person's complaints must be done before a formal diagnosis of GAD can be made.

James described himself as being a chronic worrier. Even in high school, he would often become extremely anxious several days before an exam, causing him a few sleepless nights before the test. But the worries would subside after the exam was over. Now, James was in his last year of college, and his tendency to worry became increasingly worse. Not only did he become anxious before exams, but his worries persisted afterward, as well. Socially, he had recently quit dating because, during his last few dates, his nervousness had gotten so severe that he had

1   National Institute of Mental Health (NIMH(f)). "Anxiety disorders." *NIMH website*, 2018. Retrieved from https://www.nimh.nih.gov/health/topics/anxiety-disorders/index.shtml.

to excuse himself to get sick in the restroom. During the previous year, his insomnia had increased to nearly every night, and he had additional symptoms of headaches, fatigue, and irritability. Once these problems began affecting his grades, he decided to seek help.

You can see how James's presentation is consistent with GAD, but other medical problems must be ruled out before the diagnosis of GAD can be made. For example, an overactive thyroid gland could cause such symptoms, as could the excessive use of caffeine or other stimulants. Other mental health disorders like depression can also be associated with excessive worrying. So, even if you see someone with profound anxiety and worry, the first priority is to have them assessed for other possible conditions. Once these problems are ruled out, then a diagnosis of GAD can be considered. For James, his complaints met the criteria for diagnosing GAD. The slow progression over many months and years (and his age of onset) are quite common for this disorder.

Now that you know what GAD is, what causes it? The jury is still out. Genetics, as in several other mental health conditions, does play a role. However, genes fail to give us the complete answer. Most experts believe individuals with GAD have either genetic profiles or brain chemistries that make them more vulnerable to things that normally trigger stress and worry. A number of neurochemicals (serotonin, dopamine, and norepinephrine) have been identified as potential factors in the cause of GAD.

At the same time, some other people tend to be naturally less likely to develop an anxiety disorder when it comes to stress. You probably know some people who seem to worry about every little thing and others who are essentially carefree. Applying this concept to anxiety disorders, you can appreciate how genetics may make some people more susceptible to developing GAD.

In terms of treating GAD, people often receive a combination of medication and therapy, since both have been shown to be effective. While antianxiety medications can be used to provide immediate relief when symptoms are intense, many of these medications are often limited in their use because they can be habit-forming. Instead, other medications (often some types of antidepressants) have shown great success in managing GAD. These medications adjust serotonin, norepinephrine, and other brain chemicals that in turn reduce anxiety, worry, and other GAD symptoms. Various types of psychiatric therapy, which can change a person's thinking and behavior, can also help reduce anxiety by changing how people react to different stresses.

With proper treatment and care, the vast majority of people with GAD regain the ability to function satisfactorily without excessive worry, sleepless nights, or other anxiety-related complaints. While a little bit of worry can help you be productive and prepared, too much worry can do just the opposite. Therefore, getting the help one needs when anxiety becomes chronic and extreme allows one to get back on track. If you or someone you know is experiencing a level of anxiety that is disrupting life, then it is likely time to have a professional assessment to determine if GAD may be present.

Panic Disorder

How many times have you heard people describe themselves as having a panic attack? This phrase is used all too often in everyday conversation, and in many instances, the people making these statements are not really suffering from mental health conditions. There is a difference between a panic attack and a panic disorder. To help clarify the specific features that define these mental health terms, let's take a closer look.

A significant number of people (estimated to be between 2 and 3 percent of the population) suffer from panic disorder. About six million people in the US alone suffer from this condition,[2] which affects more than twice as many women as men.[3] Given these figures, panic disorder is one of the more common anxiety conditions. By shedding some

---

2 Ibid.
3 Ibid.

light on the realities associated with this condition, you will be better able to recognize symptoms and know when evaluations are needed.

A true panic attack is a sudden onset of extreme fear that is, in many cases, associated with a fear that death or some type of significant harm is about to happen. People often feel a sense of being out of control and unable to influence when the attacks occur or their severity. Most panic attacks are associated with a number of physical symptoms, which may include chest pain, a racing heart, a pounding heartbeat, dizziness, excessive sweating, shortness of breath, tingling in the arms and legs, weakness, and/or feelings of being extremely hot or cold. Most attacks peak within ten minutes before subsiding, often occurring at any time of day or night without a trigger (they can even occur during sleep). If these are the main features of an attack, and no other cause is found (such as overuse of caffeine, stimulants, drugs, or other substances), then the event is likely a panic attack.

Panic attacks can occur as an isolated event. For reasons poorly understood, some people have a single episode and never have one again for the rest of their lives. An initial panic attack typically occurs in late teenage or early adulthood years, and this may be the only attack a person experiences. Others, however, will go on to have repeated attacks. If these recurrent episodes are associated with some other features, a diagnosis of panic disorder can then be made. The main thing that distinguishes a panic attack from panic disorder is whether the attacks are recurrent or not.

Other important criteria for diagnosing panic disorder include the presence of excessive worry or fear that another panic attack is imminent and/or evidence that the person is avoiding locations where prior panic attacks have occurred. If either of these has been present for at least one month, and the panic attacks are recurrent, then a person may indeed have panic disorder. Also, people must have some degree of functional impairment. This means they are having difficulties with relationships, work, school, or simply normal daily routines because of the panic disorder symptoms they describe. With these features present, a diagnosis of panic disorder is likely.

We cannot stress enough that panic disorder is a highly treatable mental health condition if treatment is provided early. Through various types of therapies, and sometimes with the use of medications, panic attacks and their consequences can be well controlled. But for individuals with panic disorder who fail to get treatment early, avoidance symptoms can worsen. Over time, repeated attacks can cause individuals to become more isolated, since fewer and fewer places are perceived as safe. Many people with panic disorder who fail to get treatment early may develop agoraphobia, which is an intense fear of open spaces. The development of agoraphobia, or the presence of other significant avoidance symptoms, makes the treatment of panic disorder more challenging. But for those who seek assessment early, treatment is remarkably effective.

Obsessive-Compulsive Disorder

People seem to be fascinated with obsessive-compulsive disorder, or OCD. Despite this fascination and the interest in this condition in movies and television, OCD is not well understood by most. This mental health disorder can be rather complex in its presentation. For people suffering from OCD, untreated symptoms can be quite a problem. In the US, more than two million people have a diagnosis of OCD, and many of these individuals began having symptoms when they were only children. Unlike most anxiety disorders that affect women more commonly, OCD tends to affect men and women equally.[4] On a positive note, however, once proper treatment is provided, this condition can be treated successfully. For this reason, a better understanding is needed so recognition and treatment can be given to those who need it.

What exactly are obsessive symptoms? And what is the difference between obsessive and compulsive complaints? The easiest way to think of these terms is to consider obsessions as *thoughts* and compulsions

---

4   Bhatt, Nita V. "Anxiety disorders." *Medscape*, 2019. Retrieved from https: //emedicine.medscape.com/article/286227-overview.

as *actions*. For a person with OCD, obsessive thoughts can occur in a number of areas. These may involve fears about being exposed to germs, having one's safety threatened, or having things poorly organized. Obsessive thoughts may also relate to fears about committing unrighteous or illegal acts, or to perceiving things in some bizarre way. You can appreciate how these thoughts can interfere with the ability to function normally. Often, these thoughts continually surface within the mind of a person with OCD, and an excessive amount of time is spent thinking about these things to the point where it interferes with life's responsibilities.

While obsessions are difficult, so are compulsions. Common compulsions in OCD include repeated activities involving cleaning, washing, counting, touching, or tapping. Interestingly, these actions are often done to "undo" or "negate" the obsessive thoughts. Compulsions may also involve hoarding unneeded items, repeatedly making sure specific tasks have been performed, and seeking constant reassurance from others.

Having either obsessions or compulsions does not mean a person has OCD. Symptoms of both obsessions and compulsions must be present in order to make an actual diagnosis.

> Ally, age nine, was described by her parents as having a unique personality. During the previous year, she had become overly focused on how things were organized in her room and closet. Assuming this was simply a developmental phase, as was suggested by the family physician, her parents thought little about it. But then Ally began worrying about whether the door to their home had been locked properly, and she seemed constantly worried about a burglar breaking into the house despite any known event that might have triggered such concerns. As these issues persisted (and actually worsened), Ally then developed a habit of repeatedly touching her right cheek. When her parents asked why she did this, Ally replied it somehow made her feel better.

In this scenario, Ally initially had what appeared to be obsessive symptoms related to keeping her room orderly and organized, but such features are not uncommon as part of normal childhood development. Kids often will have such phases. Her subsequent behaviors about ensuring the doors were locked, her fears of a burglar, and the constant touching of her cheek suggest a more complex problem may exist. The touching of her cheek, which sounds like a compulsive symptom, provided her with some relief. Often, such behaviors are described as making the person feel more relaxed or less anxious, even if the feeling is brief and temporary. Given the persistence of Ally's complaints, and based on the presence of both obsessive and compulsive features, she likely has OCD. With proper treatment, Ally would likely be able to return to normal levels of functioning.

In making a formal diagnosis of OCD, a doctor will often use a diagnostic scale known as the Yale-Brown Obsessive Compulsive Scale. This tool records ten different items, of which five are obsessive symptoms and five are compulsive symptoms.[5] In addition, compulsive rituals described must occur for at least one hour or more a day and result in mental distress and problems in normal daily activities. As with other mental health conditions, other causes of these complaints must also be considered and ruled out before a diagnosis of OCD can be made. For instance, OCD is commonly associated with a number of conditions including depression, alcohol and drug use, other anxiety disorders, ADHD, and eating disorders. A unique condition called Tourette's Syndrome (which has prominent features of muscle twitches and uncontrollable, erratic movements) often has OCD symptoms.[6] Evaluating for the presence of these other conditions, and an assessment for OCD itself, would be encouraged for someone presenting with both obsessive and compulsive symptoms.

When OCD individuals are taught how to adjust their thoughts and behaviors through repeated exposure to various situations,

---

5 Ibid.
6 Ibid.

improvements in obsessive and compulsive symptoms can occur. If needed, medications (most commonly some types of antidepressants) can be added to help reduce symptoms even further and allow people to regain normal functional abilities. Once again, the sooner a person is assessed, the sooner treatment can be started, which in turn allows their quality of life to be significantly improved.

Post-Traumatic Stress Disorder

You have probably heard a great deal about post-traumatic stress disorder, or PTSD. Thanks to media coverage of PTSD among military personnel after returning to civilian life, many recognize PTSD as a common problem for soldiers resulting from the traumas they experienced in combat. But combat trauma is only one type of stress or traumatic event that can trigger PTSD. Some people can develop PTSD after only hearing about other people's traumas indirectly. Because of the range of events that can cause PTSD, as well as the variations in symptoms, PTSD remains underdiagnosed. Even after a diagnosis is made, large numbers of people fail to receive treatments known to be effective. We aim to change that.

First of all, why is PTSD considered an anxiety disorder? The main reason involves the types of symptoms with which PTSD is associated. Because of the exposure to some type of major stress or trauma, people with PTSD typically develop three groups of symptoms that are all associated with high levels of anxiety.

- The first group involves what is known as reexperiencing symptoms. This is repeated intrusions of memories or images from past trauma or stress into one's mind. Such symptoms might include recurring nightmares, flashbacks, or even powerful and vivid recollections of past events.
- The second group is called avoidance behaviors. These usually involve purposeful avoidance of things that trigger memories of an event; in some cases, they can relate to feeling emotionally numb (essentially avoiding emotions altogether).

- The third group relates to being hyperaroused. Increased vigilance, irritability, and insomnia are common features within this group, as is being easily startled.

To make a diagnosis of PTSD, a doctor must explore a person's history as well as their symptoms in significant detail. To be considered as having PTSD, a person must have been exposed to some type of major stress or trauma, either directly or indirectly. Common traumas, other than military combat, often involve other forms of violence, sexual assault, physical assault, major car accidents, natural disasters, near-death experiences, or any event that triggers high levels of fear. If this history is present, then PTSD patients must also have at least one symptom related to reexperiencing, three or more symptoms related to avoidance, and two or more symptoms involving hyperarousal, and each of these symptoms must be present for at least one month. If these criteria are met, and other conditions that might mimic PTSD are not present, then a diagnosis of PTSD can be made.

It had been two years since Leslie had recovered from her physical injuries. Having suffered severely from the explosion, she was eventually told that her right leg would need to be amputated below the knee. After the initial shock, she accepted the medical facts and dedicated herself to rehabilitation. During the hospitalizations and rehab center visits, she had been somewhat shielded from the real world. But eventually, she had to return to her life and responsibilities. This was when she noted that her problems began to significantly worsen.

As a regular spectator at the Boston marathon, she had always enjoyed the crowds and the social atmosphere. Of course, that was before the terrorist attack. Now, crowds seemed to trigger intense fear within her. As a result, she had progressed to becoming a hermit in her own home.

Even the slightest noise would often provoke extreme anxiety, and images of the explosion and blood on the sidewalk forced their way into her thoughts on a regular basis. As if her insomnia weren't bad enough, when she was able to sleep, nightmares plagued her most of the time. While Leslie knew these symptoms were due to her trauma, she never thought that she might have PTSD. She simply assumed they would fade in time.

Leslie's situation is a common one (though the traumatic event she experienced is fortunately uncommon). People often develop PTSD symptoms within three months of some type of stress or trauma, but longer periods of time may pass before such symptoms develop. While Leslie's trauma was incredible, stresses and traumas of much lesser intensity can trigger PTSD. Genetics may also play a role in the susceptibility of developing PTSD. People with other mental health disorders and poor social support systems seem to be at greater risk, as well. The severity of an event does not necessarily predict whether or not PTSD may develop in any particular person.

In terms of treatment, we can report good news and bad news. Different types of therapy have been very effective in treating PTSD, such as exposure therapies, which allow a person with PTSD to be reexposed to memories of the traumatic event in a controlled manner, helping to desensitize sufferers to anxiety-provoking triggers. Therapy can also teach patients to look at memories from a different perspective and to better manage their stress through relaxation techniques. In more difficult cases, some antidepressant medications have shown benefits.

Unfortunately, there is also bad news. About one quarter of patients with PTSD refuse to participate in therapy, and another quarter drop out of therapy once started.[7] Other studies have shown that in some medical clinics, less than half of PTSD patients get treatments that

---

7   Ibid.

are available.[8] Like Leslie, many people are often never diagnosed with PTSD because they assume such symptoms are normal reactions to an event and never consider it as a possibility. From our perspective, PTSD is much more common than most people recognize. Being able to identify the common features of this disorder, and encouraging those who suffer from it to get help, is crucial in improving the quality of life for these individuals.

Knowing When to Be Worried about Worrying

Not every feeling of anxiety or worry reflects an anxiety disorder. Anxiety is a positive emotion that helps us excel in many areas of our lives. But when worries become excessive, or when anxiety symptoms occur beyond what would be considered proportionate to normal life events, then considerations for having an anxiety disorder are warranted. Hopefully, we have provided some important insights into the most common of these conditions. With this information, you should be better able to identify which worries are normal and which ones may require further assessment. As always, if concerns exist, it is better to be safe and seek psychiatric guidance. Too many people with anxiety disorders fail to get the attention they need. Encouraging the proper evaluations can make all the difference in the world in improving their lives.

---

8 Shiner, Brian, Leonard W. D'Avolio, Thien M. Nguyen, Maha H. Zayed, Yinong Young-Xu, Rani A. Desai, Paula P. Schnurr, Louis D. Fiore, and Bradley V. Watts. "Measuring use of evidence based psychotherapy for posttraumatic stress disorder." *Administration and Policy in Mental Health and Mental Health Services Research* 40, no. 4 (2013): 311–318.

Chapter 6
Psychotic Disorders

If you ask most people if they understand the term *psychotic*, most would likely respond that they do. But if you then ask them to actually define *psychosis*, in all probability, they would struggle. Why is that? After all, about 3 percent of the population will experience at least one episode of psychosis in their lifetime.[1] Though not exactly commonplace, psychosis does affect enough people's lives that some understanding of this mental health condition is necessary.

Have you ever seen a homeless man or woman on the subway talking to him- or herself in an odd way? Or standing on a corner at the bus stop behaving strangely? Chances are the person was experiencing psychosis. While these examples represent a more severe form, psychosis can present in a subtler manner, as well. This chapter will help provide a better understanding of psychosis and the mental health conditions commonly associated with it.

What Is Psychosis?
How often do you hear someone say that someone is acting "crazy"? Or perhaps they describe a person as being "psycho" or "schizo." These descriptions are vague, and often we do not really understand exactly what they mean. These loose descriptions of altered thinking are far

---

1   National Alliance on Mental Illness (NAMI). "Early psychosis and psychosis." *NAMI Website*, 2019. Retrieved from https://www.nami.org/Learn-More/Mental -Health-Conditions/Early-Psychosis-and-Psychosis/Overview.

from accurate in defining what is meant by the term *psychosis*. For example, someone might be described as "schizo" simply because they are moody or behaving contrary to what someone considers normal behavior. This alone fails to meet criteria for what would be considered psychotic symptoms. While schizophrenia is one of the most common mental health conditions associated with psychosis, many other health disorders (both psychiatric and nonpsychiatric) might cause psychosis, as well. So let's step back and take a moment to explain exactly what is meant by the term *psychosis*.

In the most simplistic terms, psychosis represents a break from reality. In order to better understand this concept, first consider how you perceive reality. Everyone, regardless of exactly what they perceive as real, uses their five basic senses to determine information about their surroundings. Your sight, hearing, and touch provide a wealth of information about things around you, as do your senses of smell and sometimes taste. Through these sensory inputs, your brain then constructs what it perceives as reality. Because most of us agree about the picture of reality our brains provide, we as a society and culture come to accept what is considered real and not real.

Certainly, some variations in our perceptions occur. For example, when asked to recall the events of a car accident, each of us will remember different details, and some of these details may even be contradictory. This occurs not because one of us has a break from reality, but because we may have focused on different sensory inputs or constructed reality in a slightly different way. These subtle variations do not reflect psychosis. Psychosis occurs when the senses are interpreted in unusual ways, resulting in a major deviation from what is considered reality.

Let's simplify things a bit further. Psychotic symptoms can essentially be grouped into two main categories. The first group, called "positive" symptoms, are the ones that tend to receive more attention. This group includes hallucinations, delusions, disorganized speech, and disorganized behaviors. Like the term *psychosis*, these terms are also often misunderstood. Having a working definition of each will help you identify what may or may not be consistent with psychosis.

Let's consider hallucinations first. Hallucinations are overt sensory perceptions that are clearly not real. For instance, psychotic hallucinations can involve seeing things that are not real (visual hallucinations) or hearing things that are not present (auditory hallucinations). Less commonly, hallucinations may involve smells, tastes, or skin sensations that are not real. Hallucinations must involve at least one of the five senses and result in perceptions that are not consistent with reality.

In contrast, delusions relate more to what one believes. When someone strongly believes something that is obviously not based on facts and is inconsistent with what nearly everyone else believes, this is termed a delusion. A person with delusions may believe that someone else is controlling their thoughts or actions or may believe they have special powers or a special relationship with God. A common delusion, called *paranoid ideations,* is when a person believes or suspects someone else is after them or has ill will toward them. A person may believe thoughts are being placed into their mind by another person (thought insertion), or that their own thoughts can be heard by others (thought broadcasting). Unlike hallucinations, delusions do not involve sensory perceptions, but relate to one's beliefs.

The other two positive symptoms associated with psychosis are disorganized speech and disorganized behaviors. If you're concerned your speech and behavior are sometimes disorganized, don't be too worried. Being poorly organized in your emails or having a messy garage is not the same thing as these symptoms of psychosis. Disorganized speech is characterized by a significant difficulty in putting ideas and thoughts together in a logical fashion. Disorganized speech might include rambling excessively, unpredictably jumping from one subject to another, and making points that have no clear association. The following list describes some common psychiatric terms that may help you understand specific aspects of disorganized speech associated with psychosis.

- **Tangentiality**—rapid changes in topics with loose (but logical) transitions without ever returning to the original topic

- **Flight of ideas**—rapid and repeated changes in subject without logical transitions
- **Circumstantiality**—lengthy talking about a topic inappropriately
- **Word salad/jargon speech**—disorganized speech in which words are put together without logical meaning
- **Neologisms**—new words created that have no known meaning

Disorganized behavior, like disorganized speech, also reflects an extreme. These behaviors are inappropriate and do not fit the situation. For instance, a person with disorganized behavior may wear winter clothes during the hottest month of summer. Or they may laugh out loud upon hearing about some tragic event. You can imagine how such behaviors are received by others. The disorganization of behaviors is such that these individuals are typically unable to complete even routine tasks throughout their day. So a clear distinction exists between being disorganized in the way we use the term every day and what is meant by disorganized behaviors in psychosis.

The second group of symptoms related to psychosis include "negative" symptoms. If you think of positive symptoms as being increased or exaggerated perceptions, thoughts, speech, and behaviors, then negative symptoms are just the opposite. With negative symptoms, a suppressed response in these same areas occurs: limited emotional expressions, reduced speech, a monotone voice, and reduced interest in activities are typical. Often a person may withdraw socially and neglect to do the things necessary for basic self-care. Reduced mental energy may be present, with motivation, initiative, and thinking often suppressed. While these features can be present in other mental health conditions, it is important to explore these symptoms if other features of psychosis are present.

Not all of these symptoms are required for a person to be considered psychotic. Different mental health conditions have different criteria regarding the type and number of psychosis symptoms that must be present in order for a diagnosis to be made. The rest of this chapter details some of these psychotic disorders further. Hopefully, we have helped you better understand what psychosis represents from a mental health perspective, so you can more easily recognize its presence.

Schizophrenia

The movie *A Beautiful Mind* portrays the life story of a mathematics prodigy as he and his family battle with his evolving schizophrenia. Presented from multiple viewpoints throughout the film, including the mathematics genius's perspective, one can gain a good appreciation for this struggle. Perhaps you already know of someone suffering from schizophrenia. Worldwide, one in every hundred people has the condition, and it strikes early. Most develop the disorder between their late teens and early thirties, men and women equally. While schizophrenia tends to become more stable after the first five to ten years, it typically remains throughout life, with full remissions being rare.[2] Understanding this condition and how to treat it is important.

What is schizophrenia? The term itself means "split mind," but despite popular media depictions, it is not some kind of "Dr. Jekyll and Mr. Hyde" condition. Instead, the most prominent features involve psychosis as it has been previously described. Many schizophrenics experience hallucinations, with auditory being more common than visual. Often, individuals will hear voices, which may tell them to act, think, or behave in a specific way that is contrary to their wishes. Many also experience delusions with paranoid ideations, thought insertions, and thought broadcasting. Disorganized speech and behavior are typically present, as well. In dealing with such an array of symptoms, it becomes nearly impossible for such individuals to carry out their normal routines.

Physics had always come easy to Bruce. He could remember in middle school how his physics teacher raved about his grasp

---

2   Frankenburg, Frances R. "Schizophrenia." *Medscape*, 2018. Retrieved from http://emedicine.medscape.com/article/288259-overview.

of the subject. With Bruce's natural interest, it was no surprise he excelled in this field and was accepted to Berkeley on early admission. Midway through his college years, Bruce became suspicious that someone was watching him. He was at the top of his class, and he suspected others wanted to sabotage his grades. Bruce also began to see his studies as being divine in nature. God had sent him to Earth for a special purpose that involved protecting the planet from an alien attack. In order to fulfill this mission, Bruce had been given special powers. In fact, he believed he had the ability to put ideas into others' minds in order to influence them. As his paranoia of others increased, he used his special powers to protect himself so his mission would not be thwarted.

Despite his efforts, Bruce's ability to keep his high class rank in school declined. His grades plummeted as he spent time on his mission. He became obsessed with others' motives, and he increasingly distanced himself from friends and family. He also began talking aloud to God, and it became clear to his friends that Bruce believed God was talking back. God even appeared to Bruce on a regular basis in the form of a bearded mystic dressed in gold. As he continued to receive divine instructions, Bruce spent more and more time in his dorm room constructing elaborate (yet unintelligible) schemes on how to build a force field around the Earth. When talking to his closest friends, he rambled incoherently about the end of times and the world's demise. But no one suspected schizophrenia until Bruce was arrested for breaking into the college's science department in an attempt to find secret documents describing the impending alien attack.

Would you have suspected Bruce had schizophrenia? Clearly, he had many features of psychosis. Yet, instead of getting the help he needed, Bruce lacked insight into his condition, and his friends distanced themselves from him as his behaviors became increasingly bizarre.

Many people with schizophrenia struggle to survive. Their symptoms and behaviors, if untreated, often prevent them from staying employed or keeping up with schoolwork. As a result, many experience poverty and homelessness. Their behaviors can often result in legal difficulties. Given these social challenges, many people with schizophrenia (at least in the United States) may no longer have health insurance by the time they are suspected of having the disorder, and this further limits their ability to be treated.

How exactly, then, is the diagnosis of schizophrenia made? In order to be diagnosed with schizophrenia, a person must have at least two of the five major symptoms (hallucinations, delusions, disorganized speech, disorganized behavior, and negative symptoms) for one month or more. At least one of the symptoms must be a "major" positive psychosis symptom (hallucinations, delusions, or disorganized speech). In addition to these criteria, a person suspected of schizophrenia must also show significant difficulties in working, caring for him- or herself, or maintaining relationships. These impairments need to have been present for at least six months. If these requirements are met, and no other mental health condition or drug use can account for the psychotic symptoms, then a diagnosis of schizophrenia can be made.

Given the complexity of this mental health disorder, you can appreciate the challenges people have when suffering from these symptoms. However, treatments do exist for many of these problems, and schizophrenia tends to stabilize over time. Ideally, treatment should target the cause of the condition, but exact causes of schizophrenia are not yet known. Genetics play a role, as family members of schizophrenics have a higher risk for developing the disorder. But this is only part of the puzzle. MRI scans commonly show that parts of the brain (the temporal lobes) are smaller in schizophrenic individuals. Many of the positive symptoms seem to result from overactivity of the brain chemical dopamine. Based on this, many of the treatments used in schizophrenia reduce dopamine activity in the brain.

While schizophrenia is not the only mental health condition that causes psychosis, it is the most common, once drug abuse and other substances are eliminated as potential causes. But recognition and treatment need to occur early. With treatment, many of the difficulties schizophrenic individuals face in life can be minimized or eliminated. New treatments with greater effectiveness are constantly being developed. By giving you information about this condition, we hope you will be better able to recognize its presence and make arrangements for professional evaluations sooner rather than later.

Other Mental Health Conditions with Psychosis

In considering psychosis, it is important to understand that it represents a set of symptoms rather than an actual mental health disorder. In other words, several different mental health conditions may have psychosis as part of their symptom complex, or a group of symptoms that occur together and characterize a disease. Though schizophrenia is a common disorder that has psychosis as a prominent feature, other mental health disorders can have symptoms of psychosis. Depression and bipolar disorder can have psychotic symptoms in some cases, as can some personality disorders. In other instances, brain tumors, dementia, head trauma, and strokes may induce hallucinations and delusions. While it is beyond the scope of this chapter for us to describe all the possible conditions associated with psychosis, we do want to highlight a few of the more interesting ones. Again, we stress the importance of seeking professional attention if psychosis is suspected, so accurate diagnosis and treatment can be provided.

Major Depression with Psychosis

Individuals with severe depression can have a break from reality—one quarter of all people hospitalized with depression are known to have psychotic symptoms. But how can you distinguish between psychosis in depression and psychosis in schizophrenia? While this can be difficult at times, some general rules exist. The person with psychotic depression must have symptoms that meet the criteria for major depression. Most commonly, the hallucinations or delusions present in major depression tend to be aligned with the person's themes of depression.

For example, delusions may involve unrealistic beliefs about a person's failures or sense of worthlessness. Or they may involve delusions about deteriorating health or death. In contrast, delusions in schizophrenia are typically more bizarre in nature. The logic used to explain delusions is usually more irrational in schizophrenia than in depression.

By using these general guidelines, accurate diagnosis is possible in most instances. Failing to diagnose and treat individuals with psychotic depression is risky. With delayed treatment, the risk for the condition to worsen increases, and the response to treatment may decline. In addition, because of the depression, these individuals may be ashamed or humiliated by their psychotic symptoms and fail to mention them during routine evaluations. Once again, it is important to have psychotic symptoms evaluated immediately.

Bipolar Disorders and Psychosis

Half of people with bipolar disorder have psychotic symptoms at some point. This figure rises to 70 percent in some groups of people with bipolar disorder.[3] One of the more challenging tasks in diagnosing a person with psychosis might involve distinguishing between schizophrenia and bipolar disorder. Imagine someone in their manic phase with rapid speech, euphoria, and racing thoughts. In addition, they have delusions or hallucinations. Dissecting the symptoms to determine whether bipolar disorder or schizophrenia is present can be difficult, but again, using specific diagnostic criteria to help identify which disorder is present provides the key.

For people with bipolar disorder, psychotic symptoms occur during the different phases of their moods. For people with Type I, psychosis may be present during the manic or depressed phases of their condition, while in Type II, the psychosis occurs during the depressed phase. When neither depression nor euphoria exists, psychotic symptoms are absent. Because mood disturbances are not the primary symptom in

---

3 Fast, Julie. "Progression of psychosis in bipolar disorder." *Healthy Place* website, 2017. Retrieved from http://www.healthyplace.com/bipolar-disorder/psychosis /the-progression-of-psychosis-in-bipolar-disorder/.

schizophrenia, these aspects help to differentiate between the two conditions. By making the right diagnosis, treatments for not only the psychosis, but also the mood disturbance, can be employed, resulting in much better responses.

Borderline Personality Disorder and Psychosis

In subsequent chapters, we will discuss personality disorders in greater detail, but for now, we can define it as a style of patterned behavior that causes individuals to have difficulties in their relationships or daily activities. Personality disorders are not uncommon, and these mental health conditions are not typically associated with psychosis. One exception to this rule is a condition known as borderline personality disorder. People with borderline personalities tend to have an inability to control their emotions well, and as a result they are often impulsive, reckless, and emotionally unstable. Relationships are routinely a struggle for people with this personality disorder. To make things more challenging, up to half may have some type of psychotic symptom.[4]

For people with borderline personality disorder and psychosis, hallucinations and paranoid delusions are the most common features. This may be difficult to distinguish from schizophrenia, but people with borderline personality disorder tend to have very high emotions associated with their delusions or hallucinations. Teasing out the details of their pasts is important to identify personality features, and some studies suggest a higher rate of childhood trauma exists among these individuals.[5] While the psychotic symptoms can be treated with medications, better long-term help can be provided through various types of counseling and therapy for the personality disorder. Because of this, making an accurate diagnosis is, as always, important.

---

4 Schroeder, Katrin, Helen L. Fisher, and Ingo Schäfer. "Psychotic symptoms in patients with borderline personality disorder: prevalence and clinical management." *Current opinion in psychiatry* 26, no. 1 (2013): 113–119.

5 Ibid.

Autism Spectrum Disorder and Psychosis

People with autism spectrum disorder (ASD) can also show features of psychosis. Children and adults with ASD have problems in communicating, poor abilities in interacting with others socially, and often repetitive movements or behaviors. People with schizophrenia can also have these same areas of functioning affected. And some ASD symptoms can be considered delusional at times. Because of this, ASD was initially called "childhood psychosis" in decades past.

More recent evidence shows a real link between ASD and schizophrenia. For example, a significant number of teens who develop schizophrenia had a diagnosis of ASD in childhood. Similar changes in brain structure and brain chemicals occur in both conditions. This has led some to suspect a common cause between the two conditions, like an early infection of the brain.[6] While this puzzle has yet to be solved, it is a good idea to explore possible ASD symptoms in childhood in a person with psychosis, since this also will guide care in a more focused way.

Making It Real

If you know someone experiencing symptoms of psychosis, you will likely be confronted with many challenges in attempting to help them. The first obstacle is in recognizing the features of psychosis. These symptoms are often subtle, and they may go unnoticed or rationalized as normal for extended periods of time. Even after medical help is sought, the road to recovery is often bumpy. Many times, people with psychosis lack insight about their problems and are unaware they are not functioning normally. This may lead to poor compliance in taking medications and keeping appointments and may also result in their refusal to be hospitalized despite significant issues. With patient rights being paramount in health care today, forcing a person to be evaluated or placed in a hospital is extremely difficult, even though it is in their best interests.

---

6   Meyer, Urs, Joram Feldon, and Olaf Dammann. "Schizophrenia and autism: both shared and disorder-specific pathogenesis via perinatal inflammation?" *Pediatric research* 69 (2011): 26R-33R.

Though challenges exist in getting the necessary care for these individuals, your support as a friend or family member is very important. With your help, ensuring that psychiatric evaluations take place is much more likely. Once evaluated, a treatment plan can be devised based on the person's individual needs. This may involve routine medications and therapy, or it may involve some of the more advanced therapies. For example, long-acting injectable medications can be used in treating patients who periodically forget or refuse to take their medications. The important thing to understand is that treating psychosis rarely has a quick solution. You can expect ups and downs, but with your encouragement and support, the ability for these individuals to function normally again is much improved.

In this chapter, our hope is that you can appreciate that psychosis implies that a person is having some break from reality. Whether their symptoms involve hallucinations, delusions, speech, or other problems, their perceptions, beliefs, and thoughts have become disorganized and irrational. While drugs may cause such phenomena, such symptoms should never be considered normal. If you believe someone is experiencing symptoms of psychosis, then seeking psychiatric evaluation for that person is a must. Not only is this important for ensuring the correct diagnosis, but it also gives them the best opportunity for early and effective treatment. This, as with many mental health disorders, offers the best chance to regain the ability to lead a normal life.

Chapter 7
Personality Disorders

How would you define the term *personality*? This can be a difficult question to answer. Each of us has different attitudes and dispositions, and we often respond to situations in different ways. Depending on your natural temperament, your experiences as a child, and even things that shaped your life as an adult, you will demonstrate your own unique personality. In our society, this means a variety of different personality types coexist at any given time. Some people react passionately to a situation, while others may react less emotionally. Some individuals are more introverted and quiet, while others are the life of the party. This is what makes our society diverse and exciting!

Think about a person in your life who tends to be annoying. Perhaps they are a little needy, or maybe they have some unusual quirks in behavior. Whatever it is, this person seems to get on your nerves and push your buttons during most interactions. Is this person just annoying? Or could this person actually have a diagnosable clinical condition known as a personality disorder? To answer that, we would need to know more details. In the rest of this chapter, we will give you some tools to help you tease those out. No one is perfect, and we all (ourselves included!) have aspects of our personalities that we could stand to adjust or change. But there are some people whose person-alities actually get in their own way in many aspects of their lives. Individuals with personality disorders often have a hard time handling daily responsibilities, integrating smoothly into their job environments, or maintaining stable relationships, simply because their personalities play out in such a way that they alienate others.

In this chapter, we will describe various traits that can be found in each type of personality disorder. It is important to remember that these individual personality traits can be found in most everyone. There are times when these traits can actually be healthy and adaptive. However, if these traits come together in maladaptive or dysfunctional patterns of behavior, then chances are the person may be suffering from a personality disorder.

Discussing each personality disorder in detail is beyond the scope of this chapter. At least ten major personality disorders currently exist, and often individuals present with a combination of different types. Therefore, we will focus on describing personality *development* as well as personality *disorders* from a general perspective, while also providing some basic information about the most common groups of personality disorders encountered in psychiatry. Through this, you will gain a better understanding of personality disorders in general and appreciate the challenges within this area of mental health.

Personality versus *Personality Disorder*

The word *personality* comes from the Latin word *persona*, which refers to one who wears a mask, such as an actor or actress.[1] Thus, the term *personality* is naturally linked to how we behave in our everyday interactions with others. In fact, the actual definition of personality refers to patterns of behavior and attitudes that people display on a regular basis over a long period of time. Various personality traits affect these behaviors and attitudes, and these combine to form one's actual personality.

If personality is defined by our behaviors and attitudes, what prompts us to behave or respond in these specific ways? As with many other mental health disorders, some experts favor genetics as a primary factor, while others believe experiences shape personality to a greater degree.

---

1   Millon, Theodore, Carrie M. Millon, Sarah Meagher, Seth Grossman, and Rowena Ramnath. *Personality Disorders in Modern Life.* Hoboken, NJ: John Wiley & Sons, 2012.

When it comes to personality, the nature versus nurture debate is alive and well. For those who support genetics, the term *temperament* is often used. Indeed, research supports a person's natural temperament as a major factor in development of some personality disorders.[2] At the same time, childhood and adult experiences also play a major role in shaping personality. Parenting styles, traumatic events, and other developmental influences have been shown to influence personality types.[3] Thus, while a precise formula describing how personality develops does not yet exist, it appears both genetics and life experiences play significant roles.

Given this information, you can easily appreciate how a large number of different personalities exist. But this hardly helps identify specific personality types. In an effort to better describe various personalities, many psychiatrists and experts have developed theories and models that attempt to describe specific personality features. Several personality tests exist that help you determine key personality traits you may have. Common areas that are considered include one's degrees of openness, agreeableness, anxiousness, conscientiousness, and extent of introversion versus extroversion. Various combinations of these five major criteria help determine your main personality type. By appreciating your own personality better, you can understand why you respond to situations the way you do.

Different personalities do exist. This diversity not only makes life interesting, but also fosters creativity and new ideas. When does a set of personality traits and behaviors cross the line from being a unique variant of normal to actually being abnormal? In answering this question, we would like to stress that the line separating the normal from the abnormal is far from solid. Instead, personality categories exist along a spectrum. On one end, normal personality styles exist where individuals are able to function well within a society. On the opposite end, personality traits result in severe dysfunctions in the ability to manage one's life. In between, a variety of combinations exist.

---

2   Ibid.
3   Ibid.

Josh was always something of a loner. His friends and family described him as a hermit, and Josh himself admitted he tended to be an introvert. Shy and content to stay at home alone, Josh rarely went out socially. Even when he went to the store for groceries, he would rarely speak to others or engage in any conversations. Josh did not fear speaking to others, but he felt little need to invest in relationships or interact with people on a daily basis. Given his personality, his job as a self-employed graphic designer suited Josh well. The contact he had with others was primarily by phone or email, and he worked from his home on a regular basis. Over time, Josh's family was concerned that he would end up alone in his old age and constantly encouraged him to get out and meet people. This was the last thing Josh wanted. Happily attending to his work responsibilities, and satisfied by spending his leisure time reading, Josh believed his life to be just perfect.

In this scenario, you might wonder if Josh has a personality disorder, but this is far from the case. Despite his desire to be alone and isolated, Josh is happy and productive in life. He has a thriving business, has adjusted his lifestyle to fit his needs, and is quite content in his daily activities. From society's perspective, Josh's introversion may be seen as odd and abnormal, but this hardly qualifies as a criterion for a personality disorder. As noted, people can have personality deficits and still not have a true personality disorder. In fact, the majority of us do have some unique personality features that others might consider unusual. Having such quirks is not enough to qualify as having a personality disorder.

While specific features of personality disorders have been described in the DSM-5 to help psychiatrists in diagnosing personality disorders, generally three key features must exist to suggest one. First, personality traits limit a person's ability to adapt well to change without significant difficulties. Second, personality traits in such individuals prevent them from responding to stress in a healthy fashion. Finally, there exists a cyclical pattern of behaviors and attitudes in such individuals that results in a progressive decline in an ability to carry out life's responsibilities.

In other words, a person with a personality disorder has difficulty functioning normally within society. This set of general criteria helps define the difference between someone who just has an outlier variant of a normal personality type and someone who actually has a personality disorder.

The identification of a personality disorder can be challenging at times. A gray area exists for what may be considered normal and what is considered a mental health disorder. For the most part, an assessment of specific personality traits, behaviors, and attitudes (along with an evaluation of a person's social functioning) allows an accurate diagnosis in most instances. Thus, if you suspect someone is struggling in life because of their persistent behaviors and attitudes, a personality disorder may be present. If this is the case, then encouraging them to be evaluated would be the first step toward improving their life.

Personality Disorders—An Overview

In this section, we would like to offer a general overview of the major personality disorders. However, as we said, going into detail about each one is beyond the scope of this chapter. Entire books have been written about each one of these disorders. In order to give you a better perspective about the various types, we will provide a brief overview of their main features and challenges.

In an effort to better appreciate different types of personality disorders, psychiatrists have grouped the various disorders into three major clusters:

- Cluster A consists of what are known as the odd or eccentric personality disorders. Paranoid, schizoid, and schizotypal personality disorders are included in this group.
- Cluster B disorders, by contrast, are considered the more dramatic and emotional personality disorders. This cluster

includes narcissistic, histrionic, borderline, and antisocial personality disorders.

- Last, Cluster C includes personality disorders that exhibit high levels of anxiety or fear. Obsessive-compulsive, avoidant, and dependent personality disorders are part of this cluster.

So that you can better grasp the various personality disorders, we will take a deeper dive into each of these clusters.

Cluster A Personality Disorders: The Odd Group

While each personality disorder has unique characteristics, grouping some together allows us to better appreciate common core features. Personality disorders within Cluster A typically have odd or eccentric personality traits as a common characteristic. This group of personality disorders shares traits that make interacting with others somewhat difficult. People who suffer from them may struggle in social situations and exhibit unusual behaviors. As a result, they are often labeled as odd, and they may increasingly shy away from people as a result. Paranoid, schizoid, and schizotypal personality disorders can all be characterized in this way. Each also shows notable features of distorted thinking patterns. Distorted thinking can range from bizarre superstitions or "magical beliefs" for individuals with schizotypal disorder to excessive suspiciousness for those with paranoid personality disorder. Individuals with any of these personality types tend to be introverted, solitary, and isolated in their daily lives. Because of these traits, the ability to function well in society may be difficult.

> William had lived alone all of his adult life and had now worked for himself for more than a decade. Previously, he had worked in a doctor's office transcribing medical dictation, but increasingly he suspected the other employees of trying to sabotage his work by purposely interfering with the taped recordings. Deep down, he felt any mistake identified in the transcriptions had been the result of their activities. When

given the opportunity to work from home, he quickly took advantage of the offer. Though others had noticed his suspiciousness, William was considered an excellent worker with great attention to detail. Despite William's being content with his isolated lifestyle, his family repeatedly encouraged him to get out, meet other people, and date. As their persistence in the matter continued, William began to increasingly suspect they wished to control and manipulate his life for their own gain. Eventually, William distanced himself further from his family and refused to seek psychological help.

In this case, William has the classic features of paranoid personality disorder. As is common to this group of personality disorders, social isolation and withdrawal are prominent features, as are disorganized thoughts. While paranoid personalities have increased suspiciousness and mistrust of others, schizotypal personalities often carry bizarre superstitions in addition to paranoid beliefs. In contrast, people with schizoid personality disorder, while also being isolated and introverted, are more commonly characterized as lacking a personality altogether. Regardless of these variations, individuals with a personality disorder in this cluster show a degree of dysfunction in their ability to interact with others and function normally in their life roles.

The personality disorders within this group tend to be quite challenging to treat. People with personality disorders within this cluster often fail to recognize they have any problems. Their ability to have insight into their personality traits in relation to their life problems is usually lacking. Therefore, convincing them of the need for therapy and change can be difficult. Particularly for people with paranoid personality disorder, any recommendations can be viewed as attacks against the individual rather than attempts to help. Despite these obstacles, therapy can be helpful as long as patience in communication and a great deal of emotional support are provided.

Cluster B Personality Disorders: The Dramatic Group

Personality disorders within this group involve personalities that are overly dramatic, highly emotional, and often erratic in their presentation. Typically, individuals with these disorders are characterized as having strong senses of entitlement and needs for attention. For example, individuals with narcissistic personality disorder present with an overly confident, arrogant, and exaggerated sense of self, while those with histrionic personality disorder show seductive and theatrical behaviors demanding attention from others. Interestingly, while narcissistic types have excessive levels of confidence that account for their behaviors, histrionic types actually have low self-esteem and use sexuality to empower their senses of self. Despite these different underlying motivations, both act in very dramatic ways in approaching life's problems. Some people with these disorders may exhibit self-destructive behaviors, even to the point of self-injury, such as superficial cutting or repeated overdose "gestures."

A great example of a narcissistic personality type can be seen in the film *Scarface*, starring Al Pacino. His character, Tony Montana, frequently ignores others' needs and concerns while pursuing his own selfish desires for fame, wealth, and power. Histrionic personalities have appeared in other films, as well. One of the more famous examples is Scarlett O'Hara in *Gone with the Wind*, as shown by her male infatuations, seductiveness, and constant need to be at center stage. These features, along with her childish behaviors and reactions throughout the film, help show how she pursues others' attention to overcome her own lack of self-confidence. Her tendency to be quite shallow and to focus on appearances and status further support her character as being histrionic.

Two other personality disorders within this cluster include borderline personality disorder and antisocial personality disorder. Both of these disorders have been shown to have strong biological bases for their development,[4] with genetics and/or natural temperament seeming to play a larger role. People with borderline personality disorder are

---

4   Ibid.

often easy to recognize. Their roller-coaster lives are characterized by rocky relationships and highly emotional reactions. Individuals with this disorder move quickly between love and hate in their relationships, and they can rapidly change their opinions of things as being good or bad. As a result, people with borderline personality disorder are often impulsive, chaotic, and disorganized, leaving a wake of destruction in their relationships as they move through life.

One of the most concerning disorders is antisocial personality disorder. Individuals with this personality type often end up in legal trouble related to criminal behaviors, as they tend to be not only self-centered and impulsive, but also socially deviant. Underlying their deviance is a basic mistrust of others, and they tend to behave in a more hostile fashion when confronted with stressful situations. These features, combined with a basic inability to anticipate the consequences of their actions, lead them into trouble quite often. This personality type has been depicted in numerous books and films over time, as antisocial personalities make for good villains in pop culture. Hannibal Lecter in *The Silence of the Lambs* is a classic antisocial personality, exhibiting marked deviant behaviors (cannibalism), distrust of everyone, and an exaggerated ego regarding his superior intellect. These personality traits contribute to his psychopathic nature and his repulsive actions throughout the film.

Therapy for this group of personality disorders can be difficult. Therapists must therefore address the presenting personality problems while maintaining a healthy emotional and psychological distance from the patients. People with narcissistic personality disorder have such inflated egos, they resist interventions that could potentially undermine their senses of self. This false self-esteem serves as a shield for dealing with life stressors. While their egos seem very strong, they are often very fragile, and encouraging them to change can be viewed as threatening to their well-being. People with histrionic personality disorder rarely seek help, and if they do, they may develop an unhealthy pattern of relating to their therapist due to associated issues of low self-esteem, dependence, and difficulty with appropriate boundaries. Individuals with borderline personality disorder, because of relationship difficulties, may seek help, but often they quit after a period of time, given their impulsive and chaotic natures. Individuals with antisocial personality disorder are challenging to treat because of their lack of adherence to social and ethical norms and basic mistrust of others. These features of these personality disorders can pose notable challenges for therapists.

Despite these challenges, therapy can provide help to many with these personality disorders, even if the benefits are limited. If a positive relationship with a therapist can be established, good outcomes can result. The use of a very specific type of therapy known as dialectical behavior therapy (DBT) has been shown to be quite effective in treating people with borderline personality disorder. DBT recognizes the tendency of people with this disorder to see things as black or white (or as polar opposites) and thus tries to change their perspective to one in which a balance is perceived between these two extremes. Through different DBT techniques, many individuals with borderline personality disorder have improved significantly.

Cluster C Personality Disorders: The Anxious Group

The last cluster of personality disorders describes those people who show high levels of anxiety and nervousness in their behaviors and attitudes. Specifically, these conditions include avoidant, dependent, and obsessive-compulsive personality disorders. The key difference among people with these three personality disorders involves how each reacts to feelings of inadequacy, low self-esteem, and stress. Different coping mechanisms are used in each based on personality traits present, and this in turn distinguishes one personality disorder from the others, despite all having some underlying level of anxiety and fear.

Let's consider avoidant personality disorder. Individuals with this personality disorder are so sensitive to others' opinions that they seek protection by isolating themselves. In contrast to persons with schizoid personality disorder who are content to be alone, often people with avoidant personality disorder actually have an intense craving for connection to others but are so sensitive to criticism that they avoid personal interactions altogether. These feelings become worse if others also criticize them for failing to achieve results. Ultimately, this leads them to shy away from social interactions. In doing so, they avoid the situation that triggers their fears and anxieties.

On the other hand, individuals with dependent personality disorder react differently to their feelings of inadequacy. Instead of avoiding social contacts, they reach out for constant nurturing and guidance from others. Individuals with dependent personality disorder often allow others to make important life decisions for them. Not only are these individuals docile and needy, they often get their loved ones around them to accomplish their everyday tasks instead of carrying them out themselves. In the process, they become helpless, dependent, and unable to accurately perceive themselves as individuals.

The other personality disorder within this cluster is obsessive-compulsive personality disorder. Rather than seeking strength from others, as do persons with dependent personality disorder, those with obsessive-compulsive personality disorder seek reassurance and comfort in rules and structure. By being overly reliant on rules and norms, they reduce their fears of the unknown. In the process, they become rigid, inflexible, and often quite demanding. These behaviors can lead to what is known as "analysis paralysis," in which the person's constant adherence to rules and structure leads to an inability to act altogether. As you might expect, this can create many difficulties in life. A character with such a personality disorder was brilliantly portrayed by Jack Nicholson in the film *As Good as It Gets*. In the film, Nicholson's character demonstrates how even the simplest things like walking down a sidewalk can be challenging as he tries to avoid stepping on cracks.

All of the personality disorders within this cluster have fears and anxieties as their common features. Some of these fears relate to the unknown, while others may involve failing to meet expectations. In trying to resolve these fears and associated feelings of poor self-confidence, the different personality types within this group approach resolutions in different ways. Each approach is pathologic and results in an inability to function adequately in life. However, on a positive note, personality disorders within this cluster tend to respond the best to therapy. Dependent and obsessive-compulsive personality disorders particularly can improve their level of function greatly with effective psychiatric treatment. This highlights the importance of recognizing these disorders and encouraging individuals with them to seek evaluation.

Challenging but Not Hopeless

In describing the various clusters of personality disorders, we hope you appreciate that treatment for many of these conditions can be an uphill battle. Indeed, some personality disorders can be difficult to treat simply because individuals may not wish to change or to participate in therapy. Many people with personality disorders choose not to seek therapy. This may occur due to a lack of insight into the cause of their problems, or therapy may be perceived as a threat to their highly delicate "stability." For those who actually do engage in therapy, a drastic event in their lives may prompt their decisions to seek help, or a new partner in a close relationship may have encouraged the visit. Extreme depression, anxiety, and other mental health problems may also develop as a result of the personality disorder, prompting a need for treatment. By the time people with personality disorders pursue treatment, significant life problems may already be present.

Despite these challenges, therapy can be helpful in many ways. Therapy allows individuals to gain insight into their behaviors and attitudes as well as their motivations. Life experiences have often helped create these tendencies, and having a degree of insight can help people make changes for the better. In addition, therapy can offer alternatives to existing behaviors and attitudes. Without this support, many people may lack the ability or resources to make such changes in their lives.

While therapy may be less effective than we want, it still offers significant benefit. In addition, medication therapy may be useful for some people with personality disorders. For example, hallucinations and delusions can develop in some people with borderline personality disorder and can be treated with antipsychotic medications. Major depression can also be associated with several different personality types, requiring medication therapy. Medications have been used in some people with antisocial personality disorder to help control behaviors.

Therapy and targeted treatments can improve people's ability to function in everyday activities, and ultimately this can help them lead healthier and happier lives. Your support and encouragement through this process is often critical to their level of participation in therapy. Not only can you help identify personality issues that are leading to life problems for these individuals, but your support thereafter is often needed to ensure that ongoing help be received. With the overview of the various personality disorders provided in this chapter, we hope you have gained a better understanding of what is meant by this term. With this understanding, you will be better equipped to get your loved ones the assistance they need to enjoy an improved quality of life.

Chapter 8
Eating Disorders

WHEN YOU THINK OF THE typical person with an eating disorder, what image comes to mind? Is it a young teenager with a skeleton-like appearance or a child with excessive obesity? Depending on your knowledge and experience with eating disorders, a variety of mental pictures could come to mind. You may know someone affected by an eating disorder, for they affect as many as 2 out of every 100 children in the United States.[1] But despite this high number, many people with eating disorders have yet to be diagnosed. This is particularly concerning because with many eating disorders, early treatment is important for positive results. For those who are not treated, complications often develop, exacerbating the seriousness of these conditions.

While each eating disorder has unique features, they all have some common characteristics that allow us to group them into one mental health category.

- Each eating disorder involves eating either excessively small or large amounts of food relative to one's nutritional needs. As a result, disturbances in both eating behaviors and weight are typically present.

---

1 National Institute of Mental Health (NIMH(g)). "Eating disorders: About more than food." *NIMH Website*, 2018. Retrieved from https://www.nimh.nih.gov /health/publications/eating-disorders-new-trifold/index.shtml.

- Eating disorders are typically associated with a distorted perception of what represents a healthy body weight and shape.
- Serious psychological, physical, and social consequences often develop as a result of having an eating disorder. Thus, all aspects of health can be commonly affected, causing difficulties in many areas of one's life.

As you learn about specific conditions in this chapter, keep in mind that each has these core features identifying it as an eating disorder.

In this chapter, we will discuss the more common eating disorders affecting people throughout the world. While these conditions were thought to primarily affect people in developed nations, increasing evidence shows that women and men in developing countries can be affected, as well. Eating disorders as a group do affect women more than men, but the imbalance is less today than it has been previously, as eating disorders among men are on the rise. Cultural minorities, previously believed also to be immune to these conditions, have been identified as being commonly affected by eating disorders.[2] By shedding some light on the various eating disorders, we hope to increase your level of awareness about these serious mental health conditions. Ultimately, this can lead to better recognition and earlier treatment so these individuals' quality of life can be enhanced.

Anorexia Nervosa

Thanks to public service announcements and the media, you have likely heard about anorexia nervosa (AN) and recognize the seriousness of this condition. This eating disorder can be life-threatening in some situations if treatment and attention are not received. Even among those treated, only half recover from their eating disorder, while 20 percent remain overly thin and 25 percent remain emaciated. Sadly,

---

2 Fitzgibbon, Marian, and Stolley, Melinda. "Eating disorders and minorities." *NOVA* website, 2000. Retrieved from http://www.pbs.org/wgbh/nova/body /eating-disorders-minorities.html.

the mortality rate for AN can be as high as 5 percent.[3] These statistics highlight the gravity of this condition, but fortunately earlier treatment offers better chances for a good response and outcome.

What is anorexia nervosa? According to DSM-5 criteria, three key features must be present. The first is a marked restriction of overall food intake, resulting in a significantly low body weight relative to a person's age and development. As a result, the ability to maintain what would be considered a normal minimum weight becomes impossible. This eating behavior is accompanied by a second key feature, an intense fear of gaining weight. This relates to the third feature of the disorder, a distorted view of what represents a normal body weight and shape. These characteristics combine to result in the actual manifestation of AN and represent the main areas where treatments are targeted.

As with any mental health condition, identifying the cause (or causes) is important, as this may offer opportunities for prevention. For AN, the exact causes have yet to be defined. In some families, AN tends to be more common, and this suggests a biological or genetic factor. However, other experts have suggested cultural causes may be important. Particularly in Western cultures where thinness, physical attractiveness, and youthfulness are highly valued, AN tends to be more common. People with specific occupations and hobbies are also at higher risk for AN, which supports a social or environmental influence. Specifically, models, actors, dancers, gymnasts, and a few others are more likely to develop AN when compared to other groups. Based on this information, it appears AN develops due to multiple factors.

Danielle was thirteen years old and struggling through that awkward stage many teenagers experience as they navigate middle school. She was somewhat shy, and unlike many of the more popular kids, Danielle often found herself alone and unhappy. If only she could be like those other girls in her class

---

3   Bernstein, Bettina E. "Anorexia nervosa." *Medscape*, 2018. Retrieved from http://emedicine.medscape.com/article/912187-overview.

who were thin and pretty, then she would have friends and be happy. But when she looked in the mirror, that was not what Danielle saw. Being what she described as "a little chunky," Danielle took matters into her own hands and began watching what she ate. She was soon skipping dinner to help lose weight, and this soon progressed into avoiding all meals and simply "snacking," as she called it. Within a few weeks, she lost several pounds and felt as if she were on the right track, but every time she looked in the mirror, Danielle still felt she had a long way to go.

Three months later, Danielle had gone from overweight to gaunt-looking. Not only were her shoulder blades and ribs easily seen on her thin, frail frame, but she had begun losing hair, and her skin was increasingly dry. Though she had already started menstruating at age twelve, her menstrual cycle had ceased. Despite these changes, Danielle still insisted she was overweight, and getting her to eat was a constant challenge. Often, Danielle was found to have hidden uneaten meals in her room or in the trash. Fearing for Danielle's health, her mother sought medical help, much to Danielle's dismay.

Danielle's story has common features and a common age of onset with people suffering from AN. In an attempt to attain a more desirable body image (albeit a distorted one), a person with AN often develops progressive health problems and an intense fear of gaining weight. Not only do they appear emaciated, but hair falls out, skin becomes dry, and both body temperature and blood pressure levels drop. For girls, loss of breast tissue and cessation of menstruation commonly occur. In advanced cases, a number of life-threatening conditions can develop, including electrolyte abnormalities, liver problems, thyroid disturbances, and even circulatory failure.

Secondary complications related to AN are very serious. Starvation diets lead to disturbances in potassium, sodium, and other electrolytes that are crucial to normal bodily functioning. A lack of adequate nutrition affects bodily hormones, which regulate metabolism, the reproductive system, and growth. It's no surprise that AN is commonly associated with serious health complications and even death. While this is concerning enough, as many as one in five people with AN attempts suicide due to related mood disturbances. It should be readily apparent that AN is not just a serious condition, but one that deserves immediate and aggressive attention.

Hope does exist for those suffering from AN. More than 50 percent of those with AN recover completely with proper treatment. However, the key to recovery involves early recognition and intervention. Individuals with longer-duration AN and lower body weight have a worse prognosis, so getting help sooner rather than later is imperative. A variety of therapies have shown promise, including individual, group, and family therapies. These seek to help educate everyone involved about the issues surrounding AN, as well as techniques to reverse the problems. While medications may play a role in treatment at times, psychological therapies are typically more effective, especially when implemented early. Thus, we would like to repeatedly stress the importance of getting help for people suspected of having AN as soon as possible.

Bulimia Nervosa

As we have said, many eating disorders share some common features, such as underlying problems related to altered weight and body-image perceptions. When comparing bulimia nervosa (or bulimia for short) to AN, it is evident that both conditions share these features as well as a fear of gaining weight. However, specific differences also exist between these two conditions. Whereas individuals with AN seek to restrict food intake to achieve their goals, those with bulimia do so by using other methods.

What criteria are used to identify someone as having bulimia? According to the DSM-5, bulimia features not only a distorted view of one's body and an intense fear of gaining weight, but also periods of binge eating during which excessive quantities of food are consumed.

Such events must occur regularly for at least three months in order to make a diagnosis, and these episodes should happen at least once a week. These bouts are also associated with a perceived loss of control over eating behaviors. After these bouts are over, individuals feel a need to compensate for their behavior through a number of methods, including self-induced vomiting, excessive exercise, the use of laxatives or diuretics, or extreme periods of fasting. This permits them to regain some sense of control, which is often needed to satisfy emotional needs.

Food binges often trigger guilt or even anxiety due to the loss of control demonstrated. As a result, the compensatory activities mentioned allow people with bulimia to appease these emotions. Regardless of the behavior chosen, the goal is to rid themselves of the excessive calories eaten in order to regain a sense of control, and to attempt to achieve the weight and body image desired. If these strategies are well disguised, parents and loved ones may never suspect a problem exists.

Like AN, bulimia occurs more commonly in women and girls, with about ten times more females affected than males. Bulimia is also a fairly common eating disorder, with about 1 percent of the population being affected over the course of a lifetime.[4] The precise cause of this disorder remains unknown. However, similar risks as described for AN also pertain to bulimia. Underlying mood disturbances, certain occupations and activities, and cultural influences likely play a significant role for many. Unlike with AN, the majority of people suffering from bulimia have either normal or excessive weight rather than low body weight.[5] At times, this may interfere with recognition of the disorder.

> Matt found himself lying on the gymnasium floor as he slowly regained consciousness. Apparently, he had fainted while performing one of his gymnastics routines, and now he found himself surrounded by his classmates and coaches. The following day, Matt's mother took him to see the pediatrician,

---

4 Hilty, Donald M. "Bulimia nervosa." *Medscape*, 2018. Retrieved from http://emedicine.medscape.com/article/286485-overview.
5 Ibid.

who took a careful history and performed a detailed examination. Despite Matt's being developmentally normal for a four-teen-year-old boy, his blood pressure clearly dropped significantly when he went from sitting to standing, and Matt noted he felt quite dizzy when performing that gymnastic maneuver. In addition, the pediatrician noted how his tooth enamel looked worn and that his parotid glands (a pair of large salivary glands found on either side of the mouth in front of the ears) were notably enlarged. These features, as well as significant facial acne and thin hair, raised some suspicions.

In exploring Matt's history further, the pediatrician found out Matt had several stomach complaints, as well. Often, Matt would tell his mother his stomach was hurting and that he was constipated and had taken laxatives as a means of improving this. At the same time, Matt admitted to vomiting on occasion when he felt bloated and full. In fact, he estimated he had done this a few times a week for the past several months. Given this information, the pediatrician shifted gears and began to explore Matt's eating patterns, thoughts about his appearance, and mood, suspecting he might be suffering from bulimia.

A bulimia case's severity is based on the frequency with which compensation behaviors occur. Mild to moderate bulimics typically have only a few of these events per week, but for more severe cases, compensating behaviors can occur once a day or more. As frequency increases, so does the risk of complications. Problems specific to bulimia involve dental problems and enlargement of the parotid glands, as noted in Matt. These abnormalities develop as a result of repeated amounts of gastric acid entering the mouth from vomiting. Other problems can include hair loss, dry skin, and acne, as noted in AN, and up to half of girls with bulimia may experience loss of their menstrual cycle.[6]

---

6   Ibid.

Finally, a number of abdominal problems can develop, ranging from bloating and pain to constipation and even vomiting blood.

People with bulimia respond well to psychological therapies, similar to those with AN. Individual, family, and group therapy techniques are typically employed, and if concurrent mood disturbances (like depression or anxiety) are present, medications may be considered. For people with bulimia, the response rate to treatment is often better when compared to those with AN, and a longer duration of symptoms does not preclude a good response to intervention. Regardless, early treatment is always preferred because this reduces the chances of complications that can be quite serious. We encourage a heightened sense of awareness for this condition and early assessment if bulimia is ever suspected.

Other Common Eating Disorders

Given the seriousness of the conditions and complications related to AN and bulimia, you can appreciate why these eating disorders receive a great deal of attention. Other eating disorders exist, some more common than AN and bulimia. The most common is actually binge eating disorder (BED). It has been estimated that anywhere from 3 to 8 percent of the population has this condition, and often BED is associated with other mental health problems. Some of the more common ones include major depression, various anxiety disorders, and even substance abuse problems.

What distinguishes BED from bulimia? After all, the name suggests individuals with BED also have binge-eating episodes, just as people with bulimia do. This is true, but the key difference is the presence or absence of compensation behaviors for the food binges. In BED, purging, excessive exercise, and other efforts to reverse the effects of the eating binges are not present. As a result, more people with BED suffer from obesity than those with bulimia, as bouts of excessive food intake lead to excess calories and weight gain.

The preferred treatment of BED involves nonmedication therapies. Nutritional counseling and behavioral therapies have been quite effective in most patients, and these can be combined with family therapy, as well. In addition to addressing eating habits and reasons for binge eating, treating any underlying mood disorders is important in helping people with this condition. Through appropriate therapies, improvement as well as recovery is often attainable in people with BED. When traditional therapies are ineffective, medications may be considered. The category of medications that has shown benefits is antidepressants, many of which have weight gain as a side effect. Thus, medications are not the primary choice for treatment in those suffering from BED.

While BED has contributed to the obesity epidemic in our country, it is not the only eating disorder that has done so. There is also a condition known as Nocturnal Eating Disorder (NED). People with NED consume large amounts of food at night, well after the normal evening meal. More than 20 percent of daily total calories consumed is usually attributed to these nighttime indulgences.[7] This nocturnal pattern of food consumption is believed to result from poor alignment of one's appetite with one's energy needs. As a result, eating occurs at night when our bodies' metabolism is typically much slower, leading to excessive weight gain.

Additional complaints from people with NED can include morning drowsiness as well as a lack of appetite in the morning hours. These features support the notion that this condition is related to some body rhythm disturbance, and not simply attributable to all those late-night fast-food commercials. Unlike other eating disorders, response to treatment in those suffering from NED is less than ideal. In many cases, this pattern of eating persists, requiring ongoing therapy to attempt a change in behaviors. However, these attempts are certainly worthwhile given the risks associated with chronic obesity.

Finally, one other fairly common eating disorder is actually better categorized as a sleeping disorder. Based on population surveys, approximately 5 percent of the population can experience this sleep-related

---

eating disorder.[8] Have you ever heard of someone sleepwalking? Well, how about sleepeating? Sleep-related eating disorder is a condition in which people eat foods at night after falling asleep. In many cases, these individuals have no memory of the event whatsoever, but they awake to a kitchen in disarray after having eaten a variety of foods. Often, the foods eaten may be actually quite unpalatable. Unlike other eating disorders, sleep-related eating disorder is due to abnormal sleep mechanisms, with sufferers acting out dreams and mental patterns in certain stages of sleep. If untreated, this condition can lead to excessive weight gain. Fortunately, medication therapies have been found to be quite beneficial in treating this condition, and thus proper treatment can effectively eliminate this unwanted eating behavior.

Mental Health for Healthy Eating

In surveying the most common eating disorders, you can appreciate that many are associated with mental health issues. For some, eating disorders reflect disturbances related to perceptions of healthy body image and weight. For others, underlying mood disturbances and mental health conditions lead to unhealthy eating patterns. In a few, both problems may exist, resulting in complex situations of altered eating behaviors. As a result, mental health professionals must identify not only the actual eating disorder present, but also any additional problems that may be complicating the situation. This allows better opportunities to treat people with eating disorders effectively.

After reading this chapter, we hope you can better appreciate not only the differences among eating disorders, but also the serious effects they can have on one's health. The most important takeaway is that early recognition is very important in allowing better outcomes for people suffering from eating disorders. For some conditions, a narrow window of time may exist for which treatment is most effective. For others, early interventions help avoid serious health complications.

---

8   Auger, R. Robert. "Sleep-related eating disorders." *Psychiatry* (Edgmont) 3, no. 11 (2006): 64.

Thus, your assistance in identifying loved ones who may be affected by an eating disorder is important. With your help and encouragement, they can get the help and treatment they need to avoid the potential complications associated with these conditions.

Chapter 9
Substance Use Disorders

YOU MAY NOT THINK OF drug and alcohol issues as being psychiatric problems, but without question these conditions fall within the realm of mental health disorders. Collectively referred to as substance use disorders, these illnesses affect millions of people in our society. This figure becomes even more astounding when one considers how profoundly a family member, friend, or loved one can be affected by the substance abuser's behaviors. We would guess that nearly everyone in our society has at some point been affected by a substance use disorder in some way. Thus, we feel the need to dedicate a chapter to this important subject in order to shed some light on this very important mental health problem.

While detailing every substance use disorder is beyond the scope of this book, we will provide a thorough overview of the issues surrounding these mental health disorders. With a better understanding of substance use disorders, you will be more able to get loved ones suffering from these conditions the help they need.

The Reality of Substance Use Disorders

Let's consider some cold, hard facts about substance use disorders in the United States. By best estimates, more than 9 percent of the US population has some type of substance use disorder. That's roughly

30 million people![1] While substance use itself can lead to a variety of health problems, these disorders are commonly associated with untimely and tragic death. Most of us can readily recall celebrities like Heath Ledger, John Belushi, and Whitney Houston, who died prematurely from substance overdoses. Icons like Elvis Presley and Michael Jackson can be added to this list. The number of deaths attributed to alcohol, tobacco, and opioids is nearly 600,000 a year. In addition, US cost estimates as a result of substance use disorders are suggested to be more than $700 billion annually due to combined direct health-care expenditures and lost productivity.[2] This is a serious public health issue in our society.

What comes to mind when you think about substance use problems? Some people may think of alcoholism, while others may consider street drugs like cocaine or heroin. In reality, substance use disorders involve a variety of substances that are used in excess and result in various functional impairments. Some substances are natural (like cannabis or peyote), while others are synthetic (like methamphetamines or LSD). Some are legalized (like alcohol and prescription medications), while others are illegal (like heroin and ecstasy). All can fall under the umbrella of substance use disorders if they meet specific criteria, which include physical, social, and/or psychological impairment.

One of the most concerning areas involves the misuse and abuse of prescription drugs. More than 50 million people will use prescription drugs inappropriately in their lifetimes, and during any given year, about nine million people will abuse these types of medications. More than half of prescription drugs abused are acquired from someone other than a health-care provider. The three most common categories

1   Grant, Bridget F., Frederick S. Stinson, Deborah A. Dawson, S. P. Chou, M. C. Dufour, W. Compton, R. P. Pickering, and K. Kaplan. "Prevalence and co-occurrence of substance use disorders and independent mood and anxiety disorders." *Alcohol Research & Health* 29, no. 2 (2006): 107–120.

2   National Institute of Drug Abuse. "Trends and statistics." *NIDA* website, 2017. Retrieved from http://www.drugabuse.gov/related-topics/trends-statistics.

of prescription drugs abused are painkillers, tranquilizers, and stimulants.[3] While all substance use disorders can pose serious threats to an individual's health, these three drug classes are especially concerning. Overdoses of painkillers and tranquilizers result in thousands of deaths each year, and withdrawal from these drugs (as well as from alcohol) is associated with high rates of death due to heart-related complications.

The DSM-5 currently recognizes several substances that may be included within a substance use disorder category. These include alcohol, tobacco, cannabis, stimulants, inhalants, sedatives, tranquilizers, hallucinogens, ecstasy, and opioids. To make a diagnosis of one of these substance use disorders, a list of criteria must be applied to a person's specific situation.[4] Altogether, nine criteria exist:

- Hazardous use of a substance
- Presence of social and/or interpersonal problems secondary to substance use
- Neglecting of major roles and responsibilities secondary to substance use
- Advancing tolerance (declining levels of mind altering or "highs" from a substance)
- Escalating quantity of use
- Repeating attempts to quit or reduce substance use
- Increasing use of time and resources to acquire substance
- Physical and/or psychological problems secondary to substance use
- Features of withdrawal from a lack of substance use

---

3   National Institute of Drug Abuse. "Popping pills: A drug abuse epidemic." *NIDA website*, n.d. Retrieved from https://www.drugabuse.gov/sites/default/files/poppingpills-nida.pdf

4   Hasin, Deborah S., Charles P. O'Brien, Marc Auriacombe, Guilherme Borges, Kathleen Bucholz, Alan Budney, Wilson M. Compton, et al. "DSM-5 criteria for substance use disorders: Recommendations and rationale." *American Journal of Psychiatry* 170, no. 8 (2013): 834–851.

If two or more of the above criteria are met, then a person is diagnosed as having a substance use disorder with the specific substance identified. Likewise, the severity of the substance use disorder is then determined based on the number of criteria met. For individuals who meet two to three criteria, mild substance use disorder is diagnosed. Individuals who meet four to five criteria are considered to have a moderately severe problem. People meeting six or more criteria are considered to have a severe disorder.[5] Through the use of these guidelines, diagnosis of substance use disorders has become more uniform, and by appreciating these criteria, you can better recognize individuals who need help, as well.

Misperceptions and Barriers

Now that you know the diagnostic criteria for substance use disorders, identifying people who need help should be easy, right? Unfortunately, it's not always so easy. Sometimes the person with the substance use problem is actually an obstacle to getting help. Denial is a common feature of substance use disorders, and justifying a need for a particular substance is quite common, too. Both those who need help and their family members often realize a person needs help only after they have hit "rock bottom." Waiting until someone reaches such a point of misery and distress to offer help is like starting to fight a fire after half the house has burned. One of our most important goals is to help such individuals and their families get help earlier, before misfortunes happen.

> Josh, a thirty-year-old sales representative, was always surrounded by friends and colleagues. Working for a pharmaceutical company, Josh actively entertained his clients. Because he had a generous expense budget, he spent nearly every night of the week taking potential clients out for drinks and dinner. After a long week of travel and entertaining, on the weekend

---

5   Ibid.

Josh felt the need to let loose. It was only natural to want to blow off some steam on the weekend, he reasoned, and Josh accomplished this by full-day marathons of beer drinking with his friends. In all his social circles, Josh was known as the happy-go-lucky guy, and the photos of him hugging someone around the neck with one hand and a cocktail in the other were too numerous to count. No one thought much of it. Josh worked hard and played hard, and he was always fun to be around.

After a few years, however, Josh began failing to meet his sales quotas, and despite his friends gradually marrying and settling down, he could never seem to keep a relationship going. He blamed it on travel and his busy schedule, but after he was let go from work for unknown reasons, he blamed it on the lack of status and money instead. Not long after losing his job, Josh suffered a string of "bad luck," including being hit by a cab one evening and fracturing his leg. He was later sued by a former friend for misleading him on a business investment. All of these pressures resulted in Josh drinking more and more to alleviate his stress. It was only when he landed in jail after two DUIs in two weeks that his family saw he had a substance use problem.

Have you ever heard someone say, "Oh, they were just self-medicating" when referring to someone with substance abuse issues? We prefer not to use the term *self-medicating* for several reasons. We believe that oftentimes the "problem" isn't really the problem—we believe that most times the *real* issue is the substance use disorder, and that the so-called "problem" has been used as an excuse to justify the disorder. Such was the case with Josh. Despite attributing his excessive drinking to an increasing number of life problems, the drinking was actually the root cause from the start. Only after he hit "rock bottom" was it obvious Josh needed help.

Certainly, various stresses can trigger substance use disorders, but the stress is not the root cause. We all have stress. In these instances, the substance use disorder has simply been revealed as a result of the stress.

Additionally, we think the term *self-medicating* legitimizes substance abuse in a manner with which we do not agree. The concept of self-medication minimizes the underlying substance use disorder and makes pursuing treatment less likely. Therefore, using a term like *self-medication* fails to acknowledge the true nature of the problem and serves as an obstacle to getting real help.

Loved ones and family members may also present as obstacles in recognizing and acknowledging a substance use problem. Codependency and enabling behaviors represent two ways in which loved ones can actually unknowingly aid and abet addictive behaviors. Just as a person using a substance excessively is dependent on that substance (physically and/or psychologically), a loved one or family member can be dependent on the substance abuser. The need of a family member to be loved, accepted, and secure is linked to their ability to care for the person who is using the substance. Therefore, and typically without knowing it, the loved one allows the reality of the situation to be ignored, making excuses for the behavior so that they may continue in a caretaker role. This never-ending cycle can result in ever-increasing dependency for the individual.

Enabling behaviors are somewhat similar, but the motivations for these behaviors may be different. For example, consider a friend who encourages someone with a known alcohol problem to go out for "just a couple of beers" to meet their own social needs. Or perhaps parents hide or ignore their own child's drug use for fear they would be embarrassed socially. Whether direct or indirect, such enabling behaviors serve to encourage further substance use and ignore the real problems at hand. In such cases, a friend or family member needs to show "tough love" instead of what they may view as nurturing love. Shining a light on the reality of the situation is what is needed, and refusing to hide, ignore, or support the behavior is a must. Only then can the magnitude of the problem be appreciated and potential help be sought.

Treating Substance Use Disorders

Substance use disorders can be complicated. Reasons for substance use vary, and addressing these issues in a specific manner helps facilitate recovery and prevents relapse. At the same time, avoiding immediate complications from the substance use is also important. Because of this, several treatment approaches are used for these conditions, and the combinations and types of interventions are tailored to an individual's unique situation. Four groups of treatments may be considered: inpatient services, medication management, counseling and therapy, and recovery support.

As most of us are aware, substance use in some situations can be associated with high-risk complications. Not only is overdose a serious concern with many substances, but withdrawal syndromes from stopping a substance abruptly can be life-threatening. In many cases, withdrawal can result in a variety of symptoms, including hallucinations, delusions, extreme anxiety, panic, elevated blood pressure, and rapid heart rates. In addition, some forms of addiction are so profound that close monitoring is needed to ensure abstinence. For these reasons, inpatient services and facility-based care exist. Whether or not these services are provided as part of an acute hospitalization, a partial hospital program, or a residential facility, each provides close medical supervision for high-risk patients.

A number of medications are used to help alleviate withdrawal syndromes, especially for substance use disorders involving alcohol, opioids, and stimulants. A number of drugs can also be used to reduce cravings of a substance or to diminish the euphoric effect a substance may provide. Such medications are commonly used for alcohol and tobacco use disorders but can serve the same purpose for a number of other substance use disorders, as well. Medications are certainly an important aspect of care for many individuals with these conditions; however, they are rarely effective in isolation.

The mainstays of treatment for substance use disorders remain various counseling and therapy services. Individual therapies seek to enhance skills in avoiding substances while pursuing healthier lifestyles and enhancing motivation for change. These therapies help individuals recognize specific stresses, situations, and emotions that may make substance use more likely. Family therapy and counseling are also used to shed light on negative behaviors such as codependency and enabling, while also teaching effective methods of support and abstinence reinforcement. Finally, group therapies combine these goals with those of peer support and acceptance. Thus, while medications and facility-based treatments seek to address short-term needs in substance use disorders, counseling and therapy strive to provide behavioral changes for long-term success.

The last category of treatment involves a variety of recovery support services for individuals with substance use disorders as well as their family members. Such services may include mentoring, coaching, education, or even self-help programs. Faith-based support programs and vocational supports are other common recovery support services. While twelve-step programs offer guidance counseling and therapies, these programs also provide extensive recovery support for substance-using individuals. In addition to providing needed assistance to help people get back on the right path, these programs provide accountability measures that are important for recovery. Family programs are also available to help people deal with substance use disorders affecting a loved one. For example, Al-Anon and Alateen offer group support services for family members and teens, respectively, whose lives have been affected by others' alcohol use. While substance use disorders certainly affect the afflicted individual, their effects can be widespread, and support for family members and loved ones is also often needed.

As you have seen, substance use disorders can be relatively complex. Because of this, treatment is likewise multifaceted and individualized. Regardless, treatments are quite effective, especially when employed early. By recognizing a substance use problem exists, and by examining the reality of a situation (as hard as that may be), you can help identify loved ones who need help and encourage them in that direction. Substance use disorders are common mental health conditions, and many barriers exist that hinder appropriate care. Applying the information in this chapter with a dose of tough love, you can better serve those you care about and get them on a road to recovery.

Chapter 10
Geriatric Mental Health

THE NUMBER OF OLDER ADULTS is increasing in America and through-out the world. From Baby Boomers entering their later years to advances in health care extending longevity of life, this segment of the population is rapidly growing. In America alone, roughly 45 million people (or 14 percent of the population) are over sixty-five, and this figure is expected to reach 100 million by 2060, compared with 16 million in the US in 1960.[1] In the last decade alone, the number of people in the US over sixty-five has grown by nine million.[2] The same trends are happening worldwide, as well. By the year 2050, nearly 1.5 billion people will be sixty-five or older, representing 16 percent of the global population.[3] Meeting these individuals' health-care needs will be an ongoing challenge.

While you may appreciate the relative aging of our nation, you may be less aware of the mental health problems affecting this segment of

1   National Institute on Aging, U.S. Bureau of the Census. "Aging in the United States: Past, present and future." *U.S. Bureau of the Census website*, 2018. Retrieved from https://www.census.gov/content/dam/Census/library/publica -tions/1997/demo/97agewc.pdf

2   Administration on Aging. "Profile of older Americans." *Administration for Community Living website*, 2017. Retrieved from https://acl.gov/sites/default/files /Aging%20and%20Disability%20in%20America/2017OlderAmericansProfile.pdf.

3   National Institute on Aging, National Institutes of Health. "Global health and aging." *NIA-NIH website*, 2017. Retrieved from https://www.nia.nih.gov/sites /default/files/2017-06/global_health_aging.pdf.

the population. More than one in five people older than the age of sixty has a mental health disorder. By the year 2050, more than 400 million older adults will need some type of mental health care.[4] While dementia and depression are the most common mental health conditions affecting this group, other conditions are also common. Suicide rates, particularly in men, increase substantially with age. Anxiety disorders and substance use disorders are also common conditions in the elderly. Geriatric mental health care is and will be a priority for us as a nation for some time to come.

Memory Loss and Aging

We all have moments when we forget someone's name or cannot recall an item on our to-do list. Some slight decline in memory and cognition is normal with aging. All too often, more advanced memory loss is attributed to aging when in fact a true underlying mental health problem exists. One such mental health problem that can cause advanced memory loss is dementia. You likely have heard the term *dementia* in relation to Alzheimer's disease, but this is only one type of dementia, although it is one of the most common. By definition, dementia refers to any decline in memory, behavior, and thinking abilities severe enough to affect daily functioning on a consistent basis. The DSM-5 now recognizes more than ten different categories of dementia based on various criteria, but all involve impairments to memory, behavior, and thinking.[5]

Overall, dementia affects about 7 percent of individuals older than sixty, but rates vary with age. For example, while only 5 percent of people in their seventies have dementia, nearly one quarter of people in their eighties are affected. Of these people suffering from dementia,

4   World Health Organization (WHO). "Mental health and older adults." *WHO website,* 2017. Retrieved from http://www.who.int/mediacentre/factsheets/fs381/en/.

5   Warchol, Kim. "Major neurocognitive disorder: The DSM-5's new term for dementia." *Crisis Prevention Institute website,* 2013. Retrieved from https://www.crisis-prevention.com/Blog/July-2013/Major-Neurocognitive-Disorder-Dementia.

more than two thirds do suffer from the specific kind of dementia known as Alzheimer's disease, which develops as a result of abnormal protein deposits being formed in the brain.[6] While the pathologic findings are well recognized in this disease, its precise cause remains unknown, and thus treatments are limited. However, there are some known interventions that can help enhance quality of life not only for those suffering from Alzheimer's disease, but also for their caregivers.

Other types of dementia include vascular dementias, in which circulation changes to the brain result in declines in memory and thinking abilities. Chronic changes can occur to the brain from long-standing blood pressure problems, strokes, atherosclerosis, and other blood vessel conditions that result in poor brain function. Thus, treating these conditions and their risk factors is important in deterring dementia in a large number of older adults. Research has shown that high blood pressure and high cholesterol are additional risk factors for developing Alzheimer's disease.[7]

How is dementia treated? The first step naturally involves making the correct diagnosis, but unless friends and/or family recognize a problem exists, the opportunity to diagnose early (when treatments are most effective) is often lost. Many quick screening tests are now available that can be performed by any health professional, and memory-screening programs (including local National Memory Screening Day programs) exist. If dementia is suspected based on these screens, then further testing may be performed in order to guide treatment. Treatments range from medications to behavioral therapies. The goal of treatment interventions is to seek to enhance memory abilities, address mood disturbances, and improve behaviors and levels of functioning. If you suspect a loved one has a memory problem, don't assume it's a

---

6   Alzheimer's Association (AA). "What is dementia?" *AA website*, 2019. Retrieved from http://www.alz.org/what-is-dementia.asp.

7   Ciobica, Alin, Manuela Padurariu, Walther Bild, and Cristinel Stefanescu. "Cardiovascular risk factors as potential markers for mild cognitive impairment and Alzheimer's disease." *Psychiatria Danubina* 23, no. 4. (2011): 340–346.

normal effect of getting older. Instead, have them formally screened so proper care can be provided.

Dementia versus Delirium

Now that we have defined dementia, we would like to introduce the term *delirium*. By definition, delirium describes a state of confusion, reduced ability to pay attention, and changes in thinking. Disturbed thinking might involve memory loss, language difficulties, and changes in perception. This description sounds a lot like dementia, and in fact, it may be difficult to distinguish between these two clinical conditions, even for medical professionals. Making this distinction is important because delirium has serious risks associated with it: the risk of death can be as high as 26 percent among older adults with delirium.[8]

What causes delirium? Many different conditions can trigger confusion, agitation, and delirium. Common causes include infections and metabolic disturbances. For instance, urinary tract infections, pneumonia, dehydration, and altered electrolytes might trigger delirium. Toxic effects of medications may result in delirium, especially among older adults. A variety of less-common conditions may be responsible for delirium, including malnutrition, liver disease, kidney disease, and neurologic conditions. However, it is important to realize that the majority of these causes are treatable and potentially reversible, so identifying the culprit is essential to reducing the health risks associated with this condition.

The easiest way to distinguish between dementia and delirium is the timing of symptoms. Dementia is a slow, gradually progressive decline in memory, thinking, and behaviors. In contrast, delirium comes on more abruptly, usually within hours to days. Thus, while both involve changes in the ability to think clearly, delirium represents a more acute and sudden change in comparison to the more chronic presentation of dementia.

---

8   Alagiakrishnan, Kannayiram. "Delirium." *Medscape*, 2019. Retrieved from http://emedicine.medscape.com/article/288890-overview.

With this basic understanding between these two conditions, let's take things a step further. Many older adults have both dementia and delirium at the same time. Of all individuals suffering from delirium, between 25 and 50 percent have an underlying dementia. In fact, dementia increases the risk of having delirium threefold.[9] This can be a bad combination. Among hospitalized elderly with dementia who also have delirium, research shows that one quarter will die within thirty days.[10] On a positive note, delirium (unlike most dementias) is a potentially reversible condition if recognized early and treated effectively. Therefore, knowing the difference between dementia and delirium is crucial to optimal care.

> Jerry's wife, Michelle, had noticed that his memory had been failing for over a year. After finally convincing Jerry to go for a routine checkup, their doctor diagnosed Jerry with early Alzheimer's disease. Since that time, Jerry had improved slightly with a memory-enhancing medication, but even so, Michelle gradually noticed Jerry was having difficulties in other areas. He no longer drove because he became confused with directions, and often he would struggle with finding the right words to say. Despite the slight decline, Jerry was still independent and able to perform all the basic activities needed. Suddenly, that changed.
>
> One evening, Jerry began insisting he needed to go to the office to handle some accounts. The only problem was that Jerry had been retired for five years. Michelle tried to convince Jerry otherwise, but despite her efforts, he continued to hold fast to his belief. Michelle also noticed Jerry actually thought it was morning instead of evening, and he would jump from one thought to the next without any real coherent connections. Michelle was able to calm Jerry down initially, but he

---

9 Ibid.
10 Ibid.

remained restless throughout the night. His restlessness esca-
lated to agitation and intense anger. Jerry actually struck out
at Michelle, but thankfully he did not make contact. Michelle
called their son over to help keep Jerry calm that night. The
next morning, Michelle and their son were able to convince
Jerry he had a doctor's appointment. Once there, Jerry was
found to have a fever with an active urinary tract infection.
Given Jerry's agitated state, his doctor admitted him to the
hospital for treatment and stabilization.

Jerry's (and Michelle's) situation is a common one. In this case, Jerry's
dementia predisposed him to having delirium, which could be distinguished from his baseline dementia due to the sudden changes in Jerry's
behavior and his confusion. Underlying infections are a common reason for such declines—the most common causes of delirium among
older adults include infections, medications, and dehydration. Among
dementia sufferers, each of these causes becomes more likely, because
these individuals are less able to care for themselves and tend to be on
multiple medications, putting them at greater risk for electrolyte disturbances, dehydration, infections, and side effects from multiple drugs.

The two most important things to stress about delirium are its
potential to be reversible when treated well and its high risk of complications. Because of these, delirium should be considered a medical emergency. Whenever a sudden mental change occurs in an older
adult, medical evaluation is needed immediately so the underlying
cause can be identified and addressed. In some cases, hospitalization
and close observation may be needed simply for patient safety while the
evaluation for the cause is being assessed. In most instances, the acute
confusion and agitation should resolve over time with proper care.

Family Issues with Dementia

Having a loved one with dementia poses many challenges for friends
and family members. The person you have come to know and love
suddenly isn't the same anymore. Bit by bit, they lose the capacity to

remember and perform routine tasks, declining before your very eyes. For this reason, the process of mourning the person you love begins well before their eventual passing, and the emotional challenges for family members can be immense throughout this time. Especially for spouses and partners, having a loved one suffer from advancing dementia can trigger depression as well as anxiety, requiring treatment for these individuals.

While you can imagine the emotional pain for anyone with a family member who suffers from dementia, the struggles for primary caregivers are even more profound. In the US, more than 65 million adults perform some type of caregiving role, and about one quarter of these individuals care for someone with Alzheimer's disease.[11] Given the demands of the caregiver role, some studies report that close to half of all caregivers experience depression. Self-reported surveys of caregivers show 15 percent reporting excessively high levels of stress, with 21 percent also reporting physical strain.[12] Thus, making sure caregivers have adequate support (and treatment when needed) is essential to avoiding this secondary complication of dementia.

Other challenges develop when a loved one has to make the tough decision of whether to place a family member suffering from dementia in a nursing home or other type of long-term care facility. No one wants to make such a decision, but circumstances may dictate otherwise. If promises were made in the past to never allow placement outside the home to happen, such a decision can be especially emotionally exhausting and fraught with guilt. Predicting the future is impossible when such promises are made, and often the time comes when it may be in a patient's best interest to be in such a facility for their own safety and well-being. Maybe you as a caregiver have reached your limit and can no longer provide the care needed. Or perhaps the person's level of

---

11 Family Caregiver Alliance (FCA). "Selected long-term care statistics." *FCA website*, 2015. Retrieved from https://www.caregiver.org/selected-long-term-care -statistics

12 Ibid.

dementia has progressed to the point at which the home environment can no longer protect them from harm.

Different scenarios exist for each family, and no single "right" decision exists. In such situations, family members and caregivers need support, guidance, and counseling to help them make the best choices possible. In addition to support and guidance from the patient's physicians and health-care providers, individual and family therapy interventions are also available for caregivers and families. Further, professional and community-based group therapies are available. In some cases, individual treatment for depression or anxiety disorders may be needed when these interventions are inadequate. Dealing with dementia is certainly fraught with an array of challenges for caregivers, family members, and even close friends. Seeking support and assistance becomes very important when faced with these extremely difficult issues.

Elderly Health Care Includes Mental Health Care

Mental health conditions in the elderly extend well beyond what we have discussed in this brief chapter. In addition to dementia and delirium, many older adults suffer from depression, anxiety, bipolar disorder, and even substance use disorders. Despite this, many are never diagnosed or treated. As a result, many function less well physically, mentally, and socially than they could.

Depression is a perfect example of a mental health condition underrecognized in older adults. Despite depression affecting up to 5 percent of the elderly in a community, three quarters fail to receive adequate care for their depression, even though most cases are completely treatable.[13] All too often, depressed symptoms are simply attributed to aging and fail to receive the attention they deserve. This is one factor contributing to the rising rates of suicide among the elderly. For men over

---

13 Centers for Disease Control and Prevention and National Association of Chronic Disease Directors. "The State of Mental Health and Aging." *America Issue Brief 1: What Do the Data Tell Us?* Atlanta, GA: National Association of Chronic Disease Directors; 2008. Retrieved from https://www.cdc.gov/aging /pdf/mental_health.pdf.

eighty-five, the rate is four times as high as the average suicide rate.[14] Neglecting mental health care for the elderly can be devastating.

These are not the only negative effects associated with inadequate mental health care for older individuals. As a group, older adults suffer from many chronic illnesses like diabetes, heart disease, and emphysema. When mental health conditions exist, the ability to properly manage these chronic conditions becomes more challenging. All adults with mental health disorders tend to utilize health-care service more than those without such conditions. Therefore, failing to recognize and treat mental health problems among the elderly contributes to unnecessary worsening of chronic illnesses and increases in health-care costs. With the information provided in this chapter, our hope is that you will be able to recognize if your elderly loved one might be suffering from a mental health condition, and if so, to seek psychiatric attention accordingly so these unnecessary problems can be avoided.

---

14 Administration on Aging, 2017.

Chapter 11
Suicide in America

YOU MIGHT THINK THAT MANY individuals who contemplate taking their own lives suffer from a mental health disturbance. You would be correct. Among all people who commit suicide, roughly 95 percent have some type of mental illness.[1] Of all the mental health disorders we've described so far, which do you think would account for the majority of suicides? That's actually a trick question. If we dig deep enough, we find that suicide is not associated with just one (or even a few) mental health disorders. In fact, several psychiatric conditions are associated with a higher risk for suicide. Depression, substance use disorder, anxiety disorders, PTSD, bipolar disorder, bulimia, and schizophrenia—all of these mental health disorders are linked to higher suicide occurrence.[2] Because of this, we will go into greater depth regarding suicide and its relationship to mental health in general.

In the US, more than 41,000 people commit suicide each year—as a cause of death, it ranks tenth overall. For individuals between the ages of fifteen and thirty-four, suicide is actually the second-leading cause of death.[3] Although you wouldn't know it from watching the news,

---

1   Soreff, Stephen. "Suicide." *Medscape*, 2018. Retrieved from http://emedicine .medscape.com/article/2013085-overview.

2   National Institute of Mental Health (NIMH(h)). "Suicide prevention." *NIMH website*, 2017. Retrieved from https://www.nimh.nih.gov/health/topics/suicide -prevention/index.shtml.

3   Ibid.

suicide is nearly twice as common as homicide in the United States.[4] Fortunately, clear warning signs are evident in many of these cases, offering opportunities for interventions that might prevent these tragic outcomes. Given the frequency of suicide, we would like to inform you about the risk factors and warning signs typically associated with suicide. In doing so, we hope to help prevent this unnecessary loss of life by giving you the information and knowledge needed to recognize suicidal risks before suicide happens.

Suicide Risk Factors

If you have had a close friend or family member commit suicide, you are aware of the extensive impact suicide can have on others. Families, friends, coworkers, and even larger communities are affected by suicide in many instances. For example, Anthony Bourdain, the well-known celebrity chef and journalist who was open about his past struggles with substance abuse recently committed suicide. Not only was his family severely affected by the loss, but thousands deeply felt the aftereffects of his suicide because of his widespread public (and beloved) presence. One question persists: how could the risk of suicide in someone so loved and so much in the spotlight not have been recognized?

A number of risk factors for suicide have been identified. Some risk factors cannot be changed—men are four times more likely to commit suicide than women. Though nearly twice as many women as men have suicidal thoughts and attempt suicide, men are significantly more likely to die from suicide.[5] Advancing age is also associated with higher suicide risk, and suicide also tends to be more common when a family history of suicide is present. Even race affects suicide occurrence, with Native Americans and white Caucasians having higher

4   Soreff, 2018.
5   McManus, Sally, Howard Meltzer, T. S. Brugha, P. E. Bebbington, and Rachel Jenkins. "Adult psychiatric morbidity in England, 2007": results of a household survey. London, UK: The NHS Information Centre for Health and Social Care, 2009.

suicide rates and Hispanics having the lowest.[6] Combine these inherent risks, and the risk of suicide becomes even greater. For people over sixty-five, white men account for more than 80 percent of all suicides.[7]

Age, gender, and race cannot be changed to reduce suicide risk. But other conditions and circumstances associated with suicide can be addressed. Having traumatic life circumstances such as incarceration or exposure to family violence increases suicide risk. Having easy access to guns similarly lowers barriers to committing suicide. People suffering from chronic disabling conditions are also at heightened risk. Common health disorders associated with an increased risk of suicide include chronic lung disease, end-stage kidney problems, multiple sclerosis, burn injuries, and HIV.[8] As noted, concurrent depression, substance abuse, and other mental health disorders also pose greater threats of suicide.

J. D. was a fifty-two-year-old police officer who had patrolled the same beat within the city for years. He had originally become a police officer as a young man after returning from a tour of military service. Early in his police career, he excelled in his role. As time passed, life experiences and the job started to take their toll on him. After a rocky divorce, J. D. struggled to adjust. He had always had a few drinks at the bar with his buddies after work, but after his marriage failed, his drinking became a nightly affair. The hazards of patrolling the inner city became progressively intense. After being shot in the right arm one evening trying to stop a burglary, J. D. began to suffer anxiety attacks. Nothing in his life was going as planned.

Over the next several months, J. D. seemed to withdraw from his friends and colleagues. He continued to show up for his shift, but once it was over, he would return home alone

6 NIMH(h), 2017.
7 Ibid.
8 Soreff, 2018.

and drink to alleviate his chronic insomnia. At work, J. D. seemed to be moody, sometimes flying off the handle for no apparent reason. Often, he would joke about "ending it all." Fortunately, one of J. D.'s good friends saw the warning signs and approached J. D. about getting some help. Because this advice came from a fellow police officer, J. D. did not resist with the typical machismo he might have otherwise shown. J. D. received counseling, as well as treatment for his alcohol use and depression, and within a few months, his outlook on life was much improved.

In this scenario, a friend astutely recognized the behaviors J. D. was exhibiting that suggested cause for alarm and encouraged him to get the help he needed. Unfortunately, this is not always the case. For some, recognizing risks and warning signs in others is difficult. Even when these signs are recognized, people who are contemplating suicide may resist help and treatment as a result of their underlying conditions, beliefs, and emotions. Thus, for family members and loved ones, being persistent while offering support remains important in overcoming such obstacles and getting individuals the proper care.

Warning Signs and Prevention

While suicidal gestures and suicide attempts can lead to opportunities for treatment, naturally suicide itself does not. Thus, in order to prevent suicide from occurring, being able to see warning signs is important. In addition to knowing specific risk factors for suicide, knowing what behaviors are associated with higher risk is similarly useful. For example, social withdrawal and isolation are often warning signs for suicide risk. Such behaviors could suggest depression, substance use disorders, or other mental health problems—these behaviors occur in many contemplating suicide. Other common warning signs may include moodiness, recklessness, uncontrolled anger, nervousness, and an inability to sleep. Individuals may be preoccupied with issues surrounding death, and they may begin giving items away, checking insurance policies, and exhibiting other preparatory behaviors. Feelings of hopelessness and a lost sense of purpose are often present.[9]

Though it may seem obvious that specifically threatening to harm one's self is a warning sign, this sign often goes ignored. Particularly if threats are communicated often and regularly, friends and family may suffer from a "cry wolf" syndrome and minimize such statements, or believe the person is "just trying to get attention." These threats and a preoccupation with death are clear warning signs for heightened suicide risk.[10] Regardless of the frequency with which such comments are made, they are red flags and should be taken seriously. Getting a loved one professional help is imperative in these circumstances, and taking such actions could make all the difference.

In preventing suicide, getting individuals proper treatment for any mental health condition they have represents an important step in the right direction. Encouraging psychiatric evaluation and treatment for depression, anxiety, schizophrenia, and other mental health disorders can reduce the risk of suicide. The same is true of substance use disorders. Alcohol, in particular, is frequently associated with depression and suicidal thoughts, since it is naturally a chemical depressant. Given the frequency with which mental health problems are associated with suicide, anyone showing warning signs and/or features of suicidal behaviors should be screened for such disorders.

In addition to these warning signs, gender-specific differences exist for how a person takes his or her life. For example, men more commonly select more aggressive approaches. Self-inflicted gunshot wounds and hangings are more common among men. In contrast, women tend to commit suicide through less aggressive manners, with medication or drug overdoses being more common. Therefore, another warning sign is behaviors in which a person seeks a means to commit suicide. A

9   National Institute of Mental health (NIMH(i)). "Suicide prevention." *NIMH website*, 2017. Retrieved from https://www.nimh.nih.gov/health/topics/suicide -prevention/index.shtml.

10 Ibid.

person inquiring about how to obtain a gun or a narcotic prescription should raise your level of concern.[11]

Unlike other medical disorders, identifying the warning signs for suicide can be challenging. Physical signs and symptoms may be less easily recognized, and emotional and mental complaints may not be shared or communicated. Therefore, being attentive to others' behaviors is important for being able to recognize the warning signs of suicide. Once these signs are recognized, proper psychiatric treatment can be provided so that prevention can be realized.

The Real Costs of Suicide

For every 100,000 people in the US, eleven will commit suicide. Recent surveys have suggested about 7 percent of all adolescents have made an attempt at committing suicide.[12] While advancing age is a known suicide risk factor, and though a greater number of older adults commit suicide than younger ones, the number of young people who die of suicide is substantial. Kurt Cobain died at age twenty-seven from a self-inflicted gunshot wound. Marilyn Monroe died at age thirty-six from an intentional medication overdose. Many other well-known individuals in the prime of their careers have chosen to end their lives. The immediate costs of such losses are certainly tremendous, but these are not the only costs.

The impact a suicide has on others cannot be underestimated. Family and friends often experience tremendous emotional and mental stress in the aftermath of a loved one's suicide, which can lead to an array of mental health issues. In addition, someone who has to deal with the emotional aftermath of another person's suicide is at a higher risk of committing suicide themself.[13] Not only does the loss involve the person committing suicide, but it also involves the loss of relationships that person had with others. Thus, the scope of the real costs of

---

11 Ibid.
12 Soreff, 2018.
13 NIMH(i), 2017.

suicide is much broader than may seem immediately apparent. This makes efforts in prevention all the more important.

By knowing the risk factors for suicide, and by being able to recognize the warning signs and behaviors that are often present, better suicide prevention can be achieved. Without question, suicide prevention can be challenging, but having this knowledge can help equip you to identify those in your life who may be at risk. This knowledge can also help you encourage proper care and treatment of preexisting mental health conditions as well as specific circumstances that trigger suicidal thoughts. As a result, you can be the difference in preventing these tragedies, which affect not only the individual but also all of their extended friends and family members.

Chapter 12
Mass Shootings

MASS SHOOTINGS HAVE UNFORTUNATELY BECOME common in society, and in the United States these events have increased significantly over the last several decades. Of all the mass shootings throughout the world, nearly one-third occur in the US. Increasingly, these attacks victimize unknowing strangers who happen to be at the wrong place at the wrong time.[1] Why do such senseless crimes against humanity occur? What provokes these mass murderers to target the innocent? Debates regarding the causes of these tragedies involve a variety of explanations, including a lack of gun control, violence on television, bullying effects, and more. From our perspective, another contributor is the lack of a cohesive and comprehensive mental health-care infrastructure in our country. In this chapter, we will shed some light on a few of the extreme cases involving untreated (and perhaps undiagnosed) mental illness and mass shootings. In the process, we will highlight changes in our nation's mental health-care system that paralleled these events.

The FBI defines mass shootings as events involving the killing of four or more individuals, but for our purposes, we will limit our focus to those occurring in a public place to distinguish from those events involving domestic violence. Using this definition, from 1982

---

1 USA Today. "Behind the bloodshed: The untold story of America's mass killings." *USA Today*, 2013. Retrieved from http://www.gannett-cdn.com /GDContent/mass-killings/index.html#title.

to 2019, there have been at least 110 mass shootings.[2] Some of these mass shooters exhibited signs and symptoms of mental illness well before the actual event. In addition, more than half of these events ended in the shooter committing suicide, which may also suggest the presence of a preexisting mental health disorder (in addition to the shooting event itself).[3] Thus, while the issues of causation and prevention are complex and involve many different levels of consideration, we strongly believe that addressing mental health issues in a more comprehensive fashion is an essential component of any effective solution.

Despite our beliefs regarding the need for better mental health care, we want to be clear about one thing: by no means are we suggesting that violent acts are caused exclusively by people with mental illness. The vast majority of people with mental health problems are no more likely to be violent than anyone else.[4] Less than 5 percent of all violent acts can be attributed to individuals suffering from mental health problems, and people with mental illness are actually ten times more likely to be victims of violence than other individuals.[5] Despite these statistics, many falsely believe those suffering from mental health issues account for a majority of violence in society today. This could not be further from the truth. Let us repeat: *Violence and violent acts are not unique to mental illness.* Violence occurs for a variety of reasons. At the same time, inadequate mental health care does contribute to some of these events. Though a small number of such events can be attributed to people with mental health problems, getting these individuals the help they need remains an important objective.

---

2   MotherJones.com. "US Mass Shootings, 1982-2019: Data From Mother Jones' Investigation." Retrieved from https://www.motherjones.com/politics/2012/12/mass-shootings-mother-jones-full-data/.

3   Duwe, Grant. *Mass Murder in the United States: A History.* Jefferson, NC: McFarland, 2007.

4   MentalHealth.gov. "Mental health myths and facts." *MentalHealth.gov website,* 2017. Retrieved from http://www.mentalhealth.gov/basics/myths-facts/.

5   Ibid.

Snapshots of Mass Shooters

When you think of a mass shooter, what comes to mind? Many people may think of an individual who was victimized or abused as a child. Others may imagine a hardened criminal with a rap sheet a mile long. While some mass shooters do exhibit such profiles, many others do not. In fact, most come from solid middle-class homes with typical American values. What triggers these individuals to become so deranged and outside the norm as to do the unthinkable? To gain a better perspective of the profile of a mass shooter, let's examine the individuals responsible for some of the most horrific events of the last couple of decades.

Eric Harris (Columbine High School, 1999)

Eric Harris, along with his friend Dylan Klebold, was responsible for the mass killings at Columbine High School in Colorado in 1999. In total, these two teens were responsible for the deaths of thirteen people and injuries to twenty-three more as they assaulted their high school with handguns while laughing aloud. Ultimately, both killed themselves after their rampage. Subsequent investigations showed the plans for the attack had been a year in the making, and the plans involved the use of pipe bombs as well as handguns. It was also noted that Eric Harris had been diagnosed years before with major depression with suicidal thoughts, and he had been prescribed an antidepressant as a result. His depression, which related in part to poor self-esteem, also included envy for his fellow classmates. Eventually, this envy transformed into hatred and rage leading up to the attacks.[6]

Seung-hui Cho (Virginia Tech University, 2007)

Seung-hui Cho was a twenty-three-year-old student at Virginia Tech University who killed two people in his dorm before mailing a personal manifesto to NBC News. He proceeded to kill an additional

---

6   Langman, Peter F. *Why Kids Kill: Inside the Minds of School Shooters.* New York: Macmillan, 2009.

thirty-two students and professors on campus while wounding seventeen others in the process. He ultimately committed suicide. In the years leading up to the massacre, Cho had been identified as a suspect in 2005 for stalking, and he was also noted to be disruptive in his college classes, exhibiting odd behavior, bullying others, and taking photographs of girls' knees and legs. He had had a prior psychiatric hospitalization in 2005. In his notes and manifesto, Cho referred to himself as the avenger of the weak and defenseless in the name of God and Christianity.[7]

Jared Lee Loughner (Tucson, Arizona, 2011)

Jared Lee Loughner was a twenty-two-year-old who planned an assassination attempt of Arizona representative Gabrielle Giffords at a political rally in Tucson, Arizona. After targeting Giffords, who suffered severe head injuries but survived, Loughner killed a total of six people and wounded thirteen others. Since high school, Loughner had been suspected of having schizophrenia due to odd behaviors. He was never diagnosed formally. He continued to exhibit odd behaviors in community college, from which he was ultimately suspended for not undergoing a mental health evaluation as ordered. In notes found after the attack, Loughner described the government's pursuit of brainwashing and mind-control techniques through the rules of grammar. After Loughner was arrested, he was diagnosed with schizophrenia and sentenced to seven life sentences plus 140 years without a chance for parole.[8]

Adam Lanza (Sandy Hook Elementary, 2012)

Adam Lanza, age twenty, is believed to have shot his mother before driving to Sandy Hook Elementary School in Newtown, Connecticut, where he then shot twenty first graders and six adults at the school.

---

7 Ibid.
8 TheFamousPeople.com. "James Lee Loughner biography." *TheFamousPeople.com website*, 2017. Retrieved from https://www.thefamouspeople.com/profiles/jared-lee-loughner-30684.php.

Police estimated he fired 50 to 100 shots total in the bloody massacre, emotionally devastating the relatively small community. Lanza was known to suffer from Asperger syndrome, a form of autism, with concurrent diagnoses of anxiety disorder, obsessive-compulsive disorder, and depression. Despite these conditions, in addition to his obsessions with mass murders and progressive social isolation, Lanza's mother had difficulty getting him the mental health services he needed.[9]

Dylann Storm Roof (Charleston, South Carolina, 2015)

Dylann Storm Roof, age twenty-one, entered the Emanuel African Methodist Episcopal Church in Charleston, South Carolina, where he attended a Bible study for several minutes before opening fire on the group, killing nine people. Based on websites Roof frequented and his own writings, it is clear that the attack was racially motivated against African Americans. As a youth, Roof had been noted to exhibit obsessive-compulsive symptoms, and he had problems with substance use, including marijuana, narcotics, and alcohol. Prior to the shootings, Roof had become increasingly more isolated and socially withdrawn, and he had dropped out of school after the tenth grade. In 2017, he was sentenced to nine consecutive life sentences without parole.[10]

* * *

In considering the profiles of these mass shooters, several things can be appreciated. For one, each of these individuals was relatively young. Most methodically planned their attacks in advance. Also, each demonstrated behaviors (and sometimes carried diagnoses) that suggested long-standing mental health problems as they struggled to behave normally in society. Indeed, mental health issues were a

---

9 Biography.com. "Adam Lanza biography." *Biography.com website*, 2019. Retrieved from http://www.biography.com/people/adam-lanza-21068899.
10 Gray, Eliza. "What we know about South Carolina shooting suspect Dylann Roof." *Time* magazine, 2015. Retrieved from http://time.com/3926263/charleston -church-shooting-dylann-roof/.

common denominator among these mass shooters, along with poor access to appropriate mental health-care services.

Explaining the Rise in Mass Shootings

You have likely heard many theories behind the rise in mass shootings. Some of the more popular ones blame poor gun control laws, parental failures, violence in the media, and the rise in bullying. In fact, politicians, activists, educators, and even celebrities voice their opinions on these issues on a regular basis, stimulating great debates. While each of these factors may indeed play a role in these horrific events and their increase in frequency, the deinstitutionalization of mental health care can also be seen as a contributing factor.

What is deinstitutionalization? Prior to the 1960s, national mental health care not only involved outpatient therapies, but it also included long-term, state-run psychiatric hospitals. These facilities (or institutions) provided a setting for individuals who needed ongoing psychiatric care. Average stays at these facilities were often five years or longer. Not only were these facilities safe places for these patients, in theory, but they may have also provided greater public safety in the process. However, because of advances in psychiatric medications, high-profile cases exposing inhumane practices at some of these institutions, and the push for greater civil rights for disabled citizens, advocates and politicians began to insist upon community-based treatment as an alternative to mental health institutions. As a result, beginning in the 1960s, long-term mental health facilities began to close state by state, and the focus of mental health care shifted to outpatient settings during the next two decades.[11]

What do you think resulted from this change? One major change was a dramatic increase in homelessness. In fact, some estimate that 25 percent of the homeless population has some type of mental illness.[12]

---

11 Fuller Torrey, E. "Deinstitutionalization and the rise of violence." *CNS spectrums* 20, no. 03 (2015): 207–214.

12 National Coalition for the Homeless (NCH). "#TBT – In celebration of mental health month." *NCH website*, 2018. Retrieved from http://nationalhomeless .org/tbt-celebration-mental-health-month/.

Another major change was a significant rise in mentally ill individuals within the prison population. In essence, prisons to a great extent replaced mental health-care facilities as institutions for a significant number of the mentally ill.

In our opinion, it is no coincidence that mass shootings have increased in number as access to mental health care and institutionalized care has declined. In 2000, the *New York Times* examined one hundred rampage killers and found that some of these individuals suffered from psychosis or other mental health problems. Despite this, these individuals typically had insufficient and/or inconsistent treatment prior to their actions.[13] Other investigations have found similar results.[14]

As the number of psychiatric institutions was reduced, the plan was to develop a comprehensive system of outpatient, community-based treatment programs in their place. This did not happen. We believe many gaps in America's outpatient mental health infrastructure therefore exist. For example, there is a lack of supervised group homes available in our communities to care for individuals needing such care; a lack of adequate financial mechanisms to fund this type of care for vulnerable groups; a shortage of mental health clinicians and professionals trained to manage this population; and gaps persist in our legal system to mandate mental health treatment in extreme situations. A comprehensive mental health-care system, one that includes effective treatment at all levels of care (including outpatient), was never truly put into place. As a result, current health-care policies and laws fall short of protecting those with mental illness and society at large.

Where Do We Go from Here?
What is the answer? Continuing to debate gun laws is not likely to dramatically change the situation. Bolstering security at every public location is simply not practical or effective. We believe the solution

---

13 Fessenden, Ford. "They threaten, seethe and unhinge, then kill in quantity." *New York Times*, April 9th, 2000. Retrieved from http://www.nytimes.com/2000/04/09/us/they-threaten-seethe-and-unhinge-then-kill-in-quantity.html.
14 Langman, 2009.

should address many key issues simultaneously, and one of these issues is developing a better mental health-care system. Parents can hardly be blamed when their child is unable to access mental health services or refuses to be evaluated. Because a significant percentage of these individuals are truly mentally ill, holding them accountable through prison sentencing does little to improve the situation. These measures fail to consider the underlying mental health problem.

Social problems require societal solutions. Currently, our mental health-care system relies on voluntary outpatient psychiatric care, but for those with serious psychiatric disturbances, these services are inadequate. Often, people with serious psychiatric disturbances don't know problems exist. Therefore, they are unwilling to go and get treatment. Inpatient hospitalization, forced outpatient care, or mandatory group home placement need to be options of care available to all. Such options allow people to get the urgent care they need, while also ensuring greater public safety.

Clearly, simple solutions to these problems do not exist. Our nation has been struggling with health-care reform for more than half a century. If we want to contribute to the solutions to mass violence, a good place to start is ensuring that mental health services are available to everyone, and mandated in extreme cases. Because many of those with mental illness struggle with keeping a job, a place to live, and needed social supports, they are also much less likely to have health-care coverage. For this reason, more expansive social programs must be considered that guarantee mental health services to anyone who needs them. With this in place, we can begin to move in the right direction.

Chapter 13
Women's Mental Health

ABOUT HALF OF THE PEOPLE in this country will experience some type of mental health disorder in their lifetime, and about one quarter can be expected to have such a condition within any given year.[1] These conditions unequally affect women compared to men. For example, anxiety and depression are known to affect women two to three times more often than men.[2] Not only do mental health disorders negatively affect the quality of life and overall health of women, but there can be significant secondary effects of these conditions on infants and children if the women are primary caregivers. For these reasons, we will identify some of the more common (and concerning) psychiatric problems that occur specifically in women.

In considering mental health problems in women, you may be aware that hormonal influences play a major role. From premenstrual syndrome to postpartum depression, mood and cognitive changes in response to fluctuating hormonal levels are known to affect a number of women. In many instances, these conditions are mild and/or transient, requiring only support and reassurance; in other situations, they

---

1 Gold, Katherine J., and Sheila M. Marcus. "Effect of maternal mental illness on pregnancy outcomes." *Medscape*, 2008. Retrieved from http://www.medscape.com/viewarticle/573947_7

2 Women's International Pharmacy. "Moods and hormones: Emotional health and well-being throughout the lifecycle." *Connections*, 2012. Retrieved from http://womensinternational.com/connections/moods.html.

become severe and have significant health risks. Women suffering from mental illness also have unique challenges in carrying out their specific roles as parents and caregivers. Failing to address these concerns can result in poor outcomes for all involved. Fortunately, much has been learned about these mental health conditions in women in recent years, in addition to their detection and management. As always, we want to emphasize the importance of early intervention, which will allow your loved ones to enjoy a better quality of life.

Mood, Cognition, and Women

You might think it strange that hormones that influence a woman's reproductive system could also have significant effects on other organ systems. These neurochemical substances have a tremendous impact on the brain's function—in fact, brain cells have more estrogen and progesterone receptors than any other organ system.[3] As a result, fluctuations in the levels of these hormones can have profound effects on several cognitive functions. In some cases, specific hormonal changes may result in beneficial effects, while in other instances, the opposite effect may occur. The complexity of these hormones' interaction with the brain is a major reason why our understanding of this mental health topic is still limited.

Estrogen has been shown to stimulate the growth of brain cells' connections and the number of chemical receptors on these cells. As a result, estrogen can enhance a variety of brain functions including attention, memory, spatial skills, and complex thought. Estrogen is also associated with improved blood circulation to the brain as well as enhanced cell repair mechanisms, which also improve thinking abilities. Estrogen is known to boost various chemicals in the brain that help brain cells communicate with one another. These chemicals,

---

3   Henderson, Victor W., Jan A. St John, Howard N. Hodis, Carol A. McCleary, Frank Z. Stanczyk, Roksana Karim, Donna Shoupe, et al. "Cognition, mood, and physiological concentrations of sex hormones in the early and late postmenopause." Proceedings of the National Academy of Sciences 110, no. 50 (2013): 20290–20295.

called neurotransmitters, affect not only our ability to think, but also our moods.[4] Given these many brain-related effects of estrogen, you can appreciate how sudden changes in estrogen levels could affect the brain's ability to perform at its best.

Though we have presented estrogen's effects on the brain in a relatively simplified manner, in reality, these effects are more difficult to predict. For example, as a general rule, too much estrogen has been associated with anxiety and tension in women. In contrast, too little estrogen typically results in depressive symptoms. More often, the most significant symptoms (such as those associated with menstrual changes and pregnancy) occur when estrogen levels go up and down, resulting in a range of mood and cognitive changes that can go from one extreme to the other. The balance between estrogen and another hormone, progesterone, also plays a part in which symptoms might occur, if any.[5] Thus, while some general guidelines can be appreciated, our understanding of the interactions between hormones and brain function still has a long way to go.

You may have heard less about progesterone than estrogen, but it is also an interesting hormone in relation to brain function. The largest number of progesterone receptors in the brain is in the area known as the limbic region. This region is important because of its strong association with moods and emotions. Therefore, sudden changes in progesterone can have significant effects on how we feel. In general, progesterone has a calming effect on mood, presumably through action on these limbic region receptors. Sudden drops in progesterone levels can often lead to anxiety and, if profound, can even lead to rage and violence. Many of the mood changes that occur in premenstrual syndrome and postpartum depression are suspected to result from sudden drops in progesterone levels.[6]

---

4   Women's International Pharmacy. "Cognition and memory: How hormones influence our minds." *Connections*, 2013. Retrieved from https://www.womens -international.com/portfolio-items/cognition-and-memory/.
5   Women's International Pharmacy, 2012.
6   Ibid.

Menstruation and Mental Health Disorders

Given the potential influence hormones have on the brain, you would expect the most significant symptoms to occur during times when hormone levels change abruptly. For women, this occurs during menstruation as well as in perimenopause ("around menopause," or the time when the female body makes the natural transition toward menopause) and menopause. Specific syndromes that are now well recognized include premenstrual syndrome (PMS) and premenstrual dysphoric disorder (PMDD). Even during puberty and around the time menses begin, teen girls often experience anxiety, moodiness, reduced concentration, and interrupted sleep. Fortunately, these mental health conditions and symptoms are better recognized and appreciated today, and as a result, women receive much better support and treatment than they did in past decades.

According to some reports, 85 percent of all women have at least one PMS symptom.[7] Fortunately, the majority of women do not require any significant interventions. By definition, PMS is characterized by an increase in tension experienced a few days before menstruation that is severe enough to affect relationships and normal responsibilities. A variety of other symptoms may accompany PMS tension, including increased fatigue, irritability, depressed mood, poor decision-making abilities, weepiness, and reduced memory. While PMS symptoms resolve completely with menopause, they often escalate between adolescence and midlife, causing significant problems for some.

A more severe form of PMS is labeled premenstrual dysphoric disorder (PMDD), which affects about 5 percent of all women of reproductive age.[8] While the same symptoms described in PMS are also experienced by PMDD patients, the intensity of, number of, and consequences from the symptoms tend to be greater. Per the DSM-5, five or more typical symptoms of PMDD must be present in order to make this diagnosis: depressed mood, anxiety, mood swings, persistent

---

7   Office on Women's Health. "Premenstrual syndrome fact sheet." *WomensHealth. Gov website*, 2018. Retrieved from http://www.womenshealth.gov/publications /our-publications/fact-sheet/premenstrual-syndrome.html.

8   Ibid.

anger, panic attacks, apathy, food cravings, sleep difficulty, fatigue, and/or reduced memory and concentration. Both conditions (PMS and PMDD) have been attributed to a relative progesterone deficiency compared to estrogen levels; some women have greater sensitivity to these changes and thus are more likely to experience PMS and/or PMDD as a result.[9]

> Cathy was about to have her thirty-sixth birthday, but she hardly felt like celebrating. Her friends had planned a night out for the occasion, but all Cathy could think about was how overwhelming it would be for her. The day before, she had begun having symptoms she knew all too well. She had become increasingly moody and irritable and had "gone off" on a bank teller for something she could hardly remember now. A sense of sadness permeated her day, accompanied by weepiness and a lack of desire to do anything. She so badly just wanted to cancel the evening and retreat to her bedroom alone.
>
> While Cathy's symptoms were certainly concerning, she knew they would resolve as soon as she began her cycle. For many years, she had assumed she had PMS. This assumption was based not only on the number of friends and family members who had commented as such, but on the change she felt each month. During the last year, the intensity of her symptoms had increased, and over-the-counter meds had not provided any significant relief. She had called in sick to work on a number of occasions because she feared how she might behave in front of her coworkers during those few days. When Cathy called her friend to cancel the birthday evening plans, her friend encouraged her to see her doctor for some help.

Cathy was diagnosed with PMDD. The number of symptoms she described, the effects these were having on her relationships and job,

---

9 Women's International Pharmacy, 2012.

and the cyclical pattern of symptoms coming and going all supported this diagnosis. She was subsequently placed on an antidepressant medication, which is a treatment for PMDD. By her next month's cycle, she had a dramatic improvement in her complaints. Antidepressants, which have been found effective in PMDD, often raise the brain's level of the neurotransmitter serotonin; some studies have shown women with PMDD have lower baseline serotonin levels. However, others support treating women with PMDD with progesterone supplements days before symptoms normally begin. This approach is also effective in many patients. Still others with milder forms of PMDD or PMS respond well to behavioral therapies that help them adapt to their symptoms.[10] Regardless of the treatment approach, the most important step is recognizing PMS and PMDD as mental health conditions so that a diagnosis can be made and treatment options offered.

You may also be familiar with changes in thinking and mood associated with both perimenopause and menopause. Here again, hormone levels fluctuate and can result in a variety of complaints. Mental dullness, general fogginess, poor concentration, and short-term memory difficulties are very common complaints among women during their perimenopausal years. Others also describe being moody, tense, anxious, and even depressed. Large research trials have examined these changes among perimenopausal women, along with their responses to estrogen. They found that oral estrogen supplements had positive effects on anxiety and depression symptoms while also improving cognition in many.[11] These findings and others support the notion that fluctuating levels of estrogen during this time are an important factor in causing perimenopausal symptoms.

Treating perimenopausal complaints involving mood and cognition is rather complex because of many variables that must be considered. While estrogen (combined with progesterone) may be ideal for some

---

10 Ibid.
11 Manson, Joann E. "Estrogen, cognition, and mood: Surprising findings from the KEEPS trial." *Medscape*, 2015. Retrieved from http://www.medscape.com /viewarticle/848794.

women, others may have conditions that make taking these hormonal medications risky. In these instances, detailed conversations with one's physician are needed in order to decide what is best for the individual situation. Other options for treatment do exist, including other medications, naturopathic therapies, and various behavioral therapies. In most cases, perimenopausal symptoms can be greatly improved if not resolved with appropriate interventions.

Pregnancy, Postpartum, and Mental Health Conditions

If you're a parent, you can appreciate the normal concerns a mother has during pregnancy and thereafter. Worries about adjusting to motherhood, being a good caregiver, and being able to physically meet the demands of those early years are all appropriate concerns for such a major transition in life. For people with existing mental health issues, these concerns can be magnified manyfold. The potential effects mental health conditions can have on both the mother and child, as well as entire families, are noteworthy during pregnancy and through the early childhood years. Therefore, we believe exploring some of the common mental health issues associated with childbearing is important.

The array of mental health conditions during pregnancy and the immediate postpartum period encompasses several disorders. Depression can occur both during and after pregnancy in a significant number of women. As many as 18 percent of pregnant women have depression during pregnancy, and more than 400,000 infants a year in the US are born to depressed mothers. Likewise, 85 percent of all women have some type of mood disturbance during the postpartum period. Conditions like bipolar disorder, psychosis, and anxiety are not uncommon for women during this time period, as well.[12] Not only can these mental health issues negatively affect women if untreated, but

---

12 Joy, Saju. "Postpartum depression." *Medscape,* 2017. Retrieved from http://reference
.medscape.com/article/271662-overview.

increasingly we are also learning about the negative effects these issues can have on infants and children.

Perhaps the most common mental health condition associated with pregnancy is the "postpartum blues." Typically, postpartum blues peak on the fourth or fifth day after delivery and resolve within a two-week period. Fluctuating moods, weepiness, irritability, and anxiety are common complaints during this time. However, unlike some other mental health conditions in this category, postpartum blues do not interfere with parenting and caregiving. Because of its mild and transient nature, long-term treatments are not routinely needed. Instead, support and reassurance usually enable women with postpartum blues to get through this difficult time without complications.

In contrast, postpartum depression is more intense and longer-lasting. Postpartum depression has been estimated to affect about 15 percent of women after delivery. This condition does interfere with maternal responsibilities.[13] Typically, postpartum depression develops within the first four months, but it can develop anytime during the infant's first year. Most women experience significant levels of anxiety in addition to typical symptoms of depression. However, women with postpartum depression are unique in some ways. Women with postpartum depression may experience intense feelings of guilt or repetitive and intrusive thoughts specifically related to their experiences of motherhood or their new infant. Intense fears regarding the infant's well-being, their ability to care for their infant, and the potential for harm for the infant are not uncommon.[14]

> Marie had long anticipated the birth of her son. She and her husband finally conceived after years of trying to have children, and now the couple held their bundle of joy with great pride. Over the next several weeks, Marie tried to adapt to her new life. At first, she appeared to make the transition well, but

13 Ibid.
14 Ibid.

gradually she seemed to struggle more and more with daily routines. She began to sleep for increasing amounts during the day and would frequently weep for no apparent reason. Her husband noticed she was no longer her jovial self, but he attributed this and her other problems to being sleep-deprived from having a newborn in the house.

Three months after the birth, Marie had become progressively "flat," showing little to no emotion about anything. Most concerning to Marie's husband was her lack of emotion in relating to their son. Marie had actually begun resenting her child for the way he had changed her life, and on more than one occasion, she had told her husband that she just did not feel like a good mom. Again, he initially attributed her feelings to being overworked and overfatigued, but after a couple of months of further decline, he insisted she tell her doctor about her symptoms. Marie was diagnosed with postpartum depression and was eventually started on medications to treat her symptoms.

As in Marie's case, a delay between the onset of symptoms and treatment of postpartum depression is not uncommon, but this delay can result in less than ideal outcomes for both mother and child. One of the greatest concerns in untreated postpartum depression involves the effects it can have on the social and emotional development of the child. Reactive attachment disorder is a condition in which infants fail to develop close bonds to their primary caregivers (usually their parents) due to the presence of neglect or abuse. Postpartum depression has the potential to not only affect immediate social and emotional attachments for the infant, but also create long-lasting difficulties in forming effective relationships throughout life.[15]

---

15 Barkoukis, Andrea, Natalie Staats Reiss, and Mark Dombeck. "Reactive attachment disorder of infancy and early childhood." *MentalHelp.Net*, 2008. Retrieved from https://www.mentalhelp.net/articles/reactive-attachment-disorder-of-infancy-or-early-childhood/.

Because of these concerns, routine screening for postpartum blues and depression should occur in the weeks and months following the birth of a child. Many effective treatments are available. For breast-feeding mothers, there are treatment options that do not involve medications, which may pose a risk to the child if a mother is breastfeeding. Individual behavioral therapies, group therapies, support groups, educational groups, and estrogen therapies may also provide great alternatives to antidepressant medications. If antidepressants are needed, selection of a medication with the safest side-effect profile can be pursued. The key to a good outcome for both mother and child remains prompt recognition and early intervention.

Pregnancy, Postpartum, and Psychosis

Managing mental health disorders associated with psychosis presents challenges during pregnancy and during the postpartum period, as well. Decisions must be made about medications being used to control psychosis and the potential effect these medications may have on the baby. Changes in the mother's weight and metabolism often require monitoring of medication dosages to avoid taking too little or too much. Ideally, discussions about having children and the risks involved should take place before pregnancy is considered. In any case, proper management of these disorders during pregnancy and afterward is important in ensuring both the mother's and infant's well-being.

For some women, psychosis may first develop during the postpartum period without any previous history of a psychiatric disturbance. Postpartum psychosis is a rare condition affecting one to two women out of every thousand, but the risks associated with this condition can be devastating.[16] Usually, and often in dramatic fashion, symptoms develop rather quickly over a few days, with increasing restlessness, anxiety, and irritability being prominent. These symptoms may then be accompanied by manic-type presentations, disorganized behaviors, delusions, and/or auditory hallucinations. If untreated, horrific outcomes can result.

---

16 Joy, 2017.

You may recall the case of Andrea Yates, who tragically drowned all five of her young children in a bathtub in the summer of 2001. Though the Yateses had their first child in 1994, Andrea's psychiatric problems didn't truly manifest themselves until 1999, after the birth of their fourth son. During that postpartum period, she began having severe depression and attempted to take her own life. These symptoms, along with delusional thinking, prompted treatment with antidepressants and antipsychotics. In late 2000, she had her fifth child, a daughter. A few months after giving birth, Andrea stopped taking her medications and deteriorated. In June 2001, she methodically drowned each child, one at a time, guided by her delusional thoughts.[17]

Andrea Yates was eventually committed to a state mental hospital after being found not guilty by reason of insanity. Despite an accurate diagnosis of postpartum psychosis by her physicians, the system failed to protect her and her children from the tragedy that ensued.[18]

Consistent with the Yates case, the risk for infanticide from postpartum psychosis is a great concern. Estimates suggest 4 percent of women with postpartum psychosis are associated with the tragedy of infanticide. Suicide is a risk in this population, as well.[19] For these reasons, women with postpartum psychosis require inpatient hospitalization for treatment, and their treatment should always be considered a medical emergency. In addition to aggressive management of this condition, safeguards must be put into place to protect both the patient and her children. Serious counseling regarding the risk for future pregnancies should also be provided.

* * *

Significant interplay between hormonal changes, cognition, and mood can occur. While these effects occur in both men and women, women

---

17 Roche, Timothy. "Andrea Yates: More to the story." *Time* magazine (March, 18th, 2002). Retrieved from http://content.time.com/time/nation/article/0,8599 ,218445,00.html.

18 Ibid.

19 Joy, 2017.

are naturally affected to a greater extent as a result of reproductive fluctuations in hormone levels throughout life. Menstrual changes over time, as well as pregnancy and postpartum periods, are notable events that are associated with potential changes in mood and cognitive functions among women. Fertility medications can have similar effects in some women. Being aware of these potential effects on mental health is thus important to improve well-being and minimize subsequent problems.

In this chapter, we have given a simplified overview of how hormonal changes influence thinking abilities and moods, as well as how they relate to specific mental health disorders. These interactions are notoriously complex, and each person has different sensitivities to these hormonal fluctuations. Genetics, past experiences, and coexisting mental health conditions all likely influence how a person will respond to these hormonal effects. Despite these variations, generalities can be made that allow us to better identify specific mental health disorders associated with hormonal changes. This in turn permits better diagnosis and care for those affected.

Chapter 14
Professional Athletes and Mental Health Issues

As a nation, we love sports. It's hard to find someone who doesn't pledge fan allegiance to a particular team in some major sport. Sports have skyrocketed over the past several decades as an entertainment product, and currently the industry as a whole earns $14.3 billion per year in the US alone. Based on recent analyses, about twenty thousand athletes and sports competitors account for these earnings.[1] These individuals are far from average in their physical abilities. What you may not realize is they are also unique in their mental health risks as a result of their profession.

Unlike other entertainment industries (such as film, television, and theater), professional athletes have a very limited career in which to showcase their physical talents. The average tenure of a professional athlete is between three and five years, depending on the specific sport.[2] Yet many are exposed to a variety of life changes and expe-

1   Burrow, Glen. "Not just a game: The impact of sports in the US economy." *Economic Modeling Specialists International website*, 2013. Retrieved from http://www.economicmodeling.com/2013/07/09/not-just-a-game-the-impact-of-sports-on-u-s-economy/.
2   Sandler, Seth. "NFL, MLB, NHL, MLS and NBA: Which leagues and players make the most money?" *BleacherReport.com*, 2012. Retrieved from http://bleacherreport.com/articles/1109952-nfl-mlb-nhl-mls-nba-which-leagues-and-players-make-the-most-money.

riences during this brief time that may be difficult to manage both during and after their careers. Additionally, compelling evidence now exists regarding the connection between head injuries and the development of various psychiatric disturbances.[3] For these reasons, we would like to bring attention to some of the unique mental health problems that often arise among these individuals and identify some of the major obstacles that may hinder them from getting the care they need.

Sports, Trauma, and Mental Health

Most people in the United States are likely aware of the relationship between sports, concussions, and mental health issues. For the last several years, mass media has exposed this relationship between head injuries and later cognitive and mood disturbances by profiling many high-publicity cases, including many professional athletes who have committed suicide as a result of their problems. The film *Concussion* starring Will Smith seeks to broaden the reach of this message even further.[4] Despite this increased awareness, our knowledge of the effects of sports head injuries on mental health remains limited. This is an evolving science, and as further investigations and studies are conducted, our knowledge will certainly deepen in this area.

The official term for concussion-related brain changes in later life is known as chronic traumatic encephalopathy, or CTE. For many decades, the medical community has been aware that boxers in particular are at risk for developing CTE later in life, even though it went by a different name (*dementia pugilistica*). Twenty percent of all retired boxers are reported to suffer from CTE based on autopsy findings.[5] Estimates among athletes experiencing concussions today show that about 20 percent will have long-term symptoms as a result of their head

---

3   Lakhan, Shaheen E., and Annette Kirchgessner. "Chronic traumatic encephalopathy: the dangers of getting 'dinged.'" *SpringerPlus* 1, no. 1 (2012): 1–14.

4   Bishara, Motez. "Will Smith: Movie 'Concussion' touches raw nerve for NFL." *CNN.com website*, 2016. Retrieved from http://edition.cnn.com/2015/12/18/sport/nfl-head-injuries-will-smith-movie-concussion/.

5   Lakhan, 2012.

injuries. CTE thus is not only specific to boxers, but also experienced by hockey players, football players, soccer players, and wrestlers. Given that as many as 300,000 concussions occur each year in football alone, you can appreciate why this represents a major concern among professional athletes.[6]

> Josh had played in the NFL for six years before he was told he would no longer be needed on the team. After several subsequent tryouts where he failed to make the cut, Josh realized his professional career as an athlete was over. As an inside linebacker, Josh had been exceptional in his skills and abilities. Willing to sacrifice his body (and head), Josh had been known for not only great anticipation of the offense's plays, but some of the most intense tackles and hits in the game. On more than one occasion, these tackles had left Josh stunned for the next several plays, and increasingly he had begun suffering from migraines and occasional dizziness. He managed to treat these with over-the-counter medicines and an occasional prescription during his playing days.
>
> After his sports retirement, Josh decided to fall back on his accounting and finance degree and opened his own accounting office. Initially, his transition went fairly well, but during the next couple of years, Josh struggled with maintaining focus and concentration. His memory became less than what it used to be, and he had trouble prioritizing his schedule. Depressed and frustrated, Josh began drinking in the evenings and on weekends to help him escape what he now called "a miserable life." When he was intoxicated, Josh often yelled at his wife and children for minor issues, for which he would then feel guilty and become even more depressed. Despite his family urging him to get help, Josh did not. Several months later, Josh was found by his wife after he overdosed on sleeping pills.

---

6 Ibid.

Although the above is a fictional scenario, a similar course of events has been experienced by many professional athletes. At least eight NFL players who have committed suicide were found to have suffered from CTE, and recent autopsies of ninety-one NFL players showed that eighty-seven had pathology changes consistent with CTE, as well.[7] While much remains unknown about CTE, symptoms commonly begin to appear eight to ten years after repetitive head injuries and concussions. Pathology examinations show an abundance of abnormal protein deposits in the brain, which are believed to result from repeated bouts of brain inflammation.[8] While identifying this at autopsy is rather clear-cut, making the diagnosis ahead of time, and preventing it, is more problematic.

What are the early signs of CTE in athletes? Initially, headaches and reduced ability to pay attention and concentrate are most common. In time, these symptoms are accompanied by short-term memory loss, along with mood changes such as depression and explosiveness. As CTE advances, cognitive abilities decline even further, leading to dementia along with aggressiveness, language disturbances, and a variety of abnormal movements. As with Josh, many individuals suffering from CTE also begin using drugs and alcohol to cope with their mental health problems. Suicide attempts are not uncommon.

While specific treatments are not yet available to reverse the effects of recurrent head traumas and halt CTE progression, proactive and preventive efforts are underway to reduce its occurrence. As mental health professionals, we believe the benefits of prevention are most effective currently, but at the same time, early recognition offers opportunities to provide medical and behavioral supports to reduce symptom severity and hopefully avoid some of the worst complications.

Sports and Gambling

Substance abuse and addictions are not uncommon for some professional athletes in dealing with the pressures associated with their

---

7   Bishara, 2016.

8   Lakhan, 2012.

roles. Likewise, substance use among athletes with CTE has already been noted as common. There are other addictions that tend to be more prevalent among athletes when compared to the rest of the population—specifically, addictions to gambling.[9] While you are likely aware of some of the high-profile athletes with gambling problems, you may not appreciate how common this behavior actually is among many athletes.

Gambling addiction, known as compulsive gambling disorder, represents a problem with impulse control. In other words, despite telltale signs of a gambling problem, individuals cannot control their behavior, and they repeatedly choose to gamble over and over again. Compulsive gambling affects between 2 and 4 percent of the general population,[10] but the actual rates of occurrence among professional athletes are not well known. Based on a number of surveys, however, these figures are suspected of being much higher. In a recent ESPN poll of professional athletes, more than half gambled on nonsports items, while one third gambled on sports unrelated to their own.[11] Student athletes in college show similar figures, with 45 percent gambling on sports on a regular basis and 5 percent reporting that they provided inside information, bet on a game in which they participated, and/or accepted money for performing poorly in a game.[12] Gambling on sports and other activities, including sporting events in which an athlete may participate, does not necessarily indicate a compulsive gambling problem. However, these

9   St-Pierre, Renée A., Caroline E. Temcheff, Rina Gupta, Jeffrey Derevensky, and Thomas S. Paskus. "Predicting gambling problems from gambling outcome expectancies in college student-athletes." *Journal of Gambling Studies* 30, no. 1 (2014): 47–60.

10 PsychCentral Staff. "Pathological gambling symptoms." *PsychCentral website*, 2018. Retrieved from http://psychcentral.com/disorders/pathological-gambling -symptoms/.

11 Sports Illustrated Wire. "ESPN poll: 63 percent of pro athletes think sports betting should be legal." *Sports Illustrated website*, 2015. Retrieved from http://www.si.com /more-sports/2015/02/05/espn-poll-pro-athletes-majority-legal-sports-betting.

12 Shead, N. Will, Jeffrey L. Derevensky, and Thomas S. Paskus. "Trends in gambling behavior among college student-athletes: A comparison of 2004 and 2008 NCAA survey data." *Journal of Gambling Issues* (2014): 1–21.

statistics are noteworthy in that a percentage of these individuals will suffer from a gambling addiction.

Like other impulse-control disorders, compulsive gambling represents a destructive problem for professional athletes and their loved ones. The behavior is personally destructive emotionally, mentally, and financially; gambling behavior also risks the athlete's eligibility in sports participation and compromises the integrity of the games in general. Pete Rose, who reportedly bet on fifty-two Cincinnati Reds baseball games in 1987 while managing the team, is the most infamous example of this phenomenon. He reportedly bet more than $10,000 a day on the games. As a consequence of his actions, he has been banned from the sport for life. Other notable examples include Charles Barkley (former NBA star with estimated losses of more than $10 million), John Daly (professional golfer who lost $55 million between 1991 and 2007), and even Michael Jordan (arguably one of the best players to ever play in the NBA).[13]

> Trey had loved sports since the moment he had been able to walk, and throughout his childhood, he had participated in all the major sports. As he grew older, he was forced to narrow down his choice of which sport he wanted to play. Ultimately, he chose hockey. Despite dedicating his life to hockey, he continued to stay involved with other sports. He loved his fantasy football and basketball leagues, and he remained an avid baseball fan. Once he got into college, where he was given a scholarship to play hockey, his buddies encouraged Trey to wager on some of the other sports for fun. He found it exhilarating. Because he knew so much about the games, he assumed it was a great chance to make some much-needed cash.
>
> Trey didn't do quite as well as he had hoped while gambling during college, but the thrill of winning a bet drove him

---

13 Ackerman, McArton. "8 pro-athletes with outrageous gambling addictions." Rehab.com, June 6th, 2014. Retrieved from http://www.rehabs.com/8-pro-athletes -with-outrageous-gambling-addictions/.

to continue to wager periodically. Once he was signed to an NHL team after college and money became less of a concern, he began to indulge even more in various types of gambling. Trey not only bet on sports now, but he also frequented casinos while on the road and arranged at least three trips a year to Las Vegas. Trey's wagers (and losses) grew in size, but he always knew the "big win" that would make everything right was just around the corner. Three years later, despite having advanced to a six-figure salary in the NHL, Trey found himself in serious debt and serious trouble. Not only had he squandered the money he had earned, but his credit was maxed and his close friends had distanced themselves from him.

How do you know if someone has a compulsive gambling condition? Categorically, as outlined in the DSM-5, individuals with this disorder exhibit some common features:

- Preoccupation with gambling activities
- Tolerance with escalating amounts gambled
- Loss of control in trying to quit
- Withdrawal symptoms when not gambling
- Escape to gambling to enhance mood
- Increase of gambling to chase debts and losses
- Lies told to others about gambling amounts or problems
- Involvement in illegal activities to finance gambling
- Relationships put at risk for gambling
- Bailouts sought from others for gambling debts

Individuals must have five or more of these symptoms in order to be formally diagnosed with a compulsive gambling problem.

While compulsive gambling is a serious problem for anyone, its impact on the lives of professional athletes can be even more profound. In part, this stems from the fact that sports is their livelihood, but the limited duration of income earnings from sports for many athletes also plays a role. Even for a brief period of time, for professional athletes, compulsive gambling can erase financial savings and hinder future earnings, resulting in lifetime effects. Because of this and the exposure of athletes to sports gambling specifically, preventive education and counseling is supported by many professional sports leagues today. Once diagnosed, aggressive treatment through individual, family, and group behavioral therapies is needed.

I'm Retired from Sports . . . Now What?

What happens when you go from being paid millions of dollars, receiving the adoration of screaming sports fans, and being in the media spotlight to being a regular member of society? While not every professional athlete fits into this category, many do, and dealing with such a major transition can be challenging and lead to a variety of mental health problems. Some of us have experienced some type of transition, such as going from a most-valued employee to a supportive role for a company. For professional athletes, a supportive role (like coaching or sports media) may not be available, and the magnitude of the fame, wealth, and power lost is substantial. For these reasons, retiring athletes can struggle with this life transition.

Generally, three major areas of concern exist for retiring professional athletes. The first is the emotional stress related to making the day-to-day adjustments to a more average lifestyle. Most athletes at this level have dedicated tremendous amounts of time, energy, and resources to achieving their superior physical abilities. No longer having a stage upon which to showcase these talents triggers a mourning process that is accompanied by all the typical emotions associated with loss. Denial, anger, frustration, and many other emotional experiences result, and these can cause anxiety and depression in some athletes. Anticipating, as well as identifying, such emotional reactions is important in trying to alleviate these symptoms and in facilitating a more normal transition.

A second major area of stress is financial security. While you may have a perception that professional athletes make large salaries (and they do), the length of time such compensation is provided is very limited. Particularly for athletes who do not have secondary careers upon which to rely, the sudden loss of income can be devastating unless proper planning has occurred. Unfortunately, for many young athletes, money is squandered on lavish lifestyles during the peak of their fame, leaving little if any financial resources when their retirement from sports arrives. As a major source of life stress, this can trigger a variety of problems, including substance use, depression, and anxiety. Thus, appreciating this risk for professional athletes ahead of time is important.

The final major area of concern is a common condition among retired athletes: chronic pain. Particularly in contact sports, chronic pain is an enduring problem for many athletes, requiring some type of pain management. Chronic pain can of course lead to many mental health problems. In addition to limiting activities and causing sleep difficulties, long-standing pain is associated with higher rates of depression as well as higher occurrences of substance abuse. Along with secondary mental health problems, chronic pain can also lead to relationship problems, further limiting support for these athletes.

Overall, retirement pressures and their effects on professional athletes differ in many ways from the retirement pressures other individuals may face. The intensity of these pressures can be overwhelming, particularly if an athlete was placed in the limelight and enjoyed the fame and wealth associated with it. Many professional sports leagues now have programs to educate athletes about these pressures, which has helped reduced the frequency of mental health problems after retirement. But these mental health problems still occur in a number of professional athletes, and being aware of the risks for developing such conditions can help get an athlete help sooner rather than later and help them avoid more serious problems.

A Final Thought about Sports and Mental Health

Hopefully, you can appreciate the special mental health challenges professional athletes might experience based on their unique situations. Concussions, gambling, and early retirement issues can each result in mental health problems for many, requiring ongoing psychiatric care. For both male and female athletes, a stigma exists about mental health conditions. In many sports cultures, having a mental health disorder is perceived as an inherent weakness—and weakness, in almost all circumstances, is believed to be contrary to sports excellence. This stigma associated with mental health conditions among athletes represents a serious barrier to both diagnosis and treatment.

In recent years, some high-profile professional athletes have become advocates for erasing such stigmas surrounding mental health disorders. Brandon Marshall, a well-known NFL wide receiver, has invested significant energy and money into raising awareness about the prevalence of mental health problems among athletes and the treatment barriers that exist for them. As someone with borderline personality disorder, Marshall has firsthand experience with biases and prejudices related to individuals who might have a mental health disorder. Slowly but progressively, his nonprofit organization, Project Borderline, is making strides in this regard.[14]

While mental health disorders may be perceived with bias throughout society, this stigma is more prevalent within the sports community because of the nature of its culture. Physical injuries are appreciated because they are tangible and usually obvious, but mental health injuries are not. Instead of being viewed as a need for help, they are often perceived as a sign of mental weakness. This directly conflicts with the concept that mental toughness is needed to excel in professional sports, which is preached at every level of athletic participation. Fortunately, greater awareness of mental health problems related to concussions has helped to reduce this stigma. Our hope is that in time, this will allow all professional athletes to get the help they need without fear of their athletic abilities being questioned.

---

14 Project 375. "About us: Who we are." *Project 375 website*, 2017. Retrieved from https://project375.org/about-us/who-we-are/.

Conclusion

IMAGINE FOR A MOMENT YOU are walking down the sidewalk on your way to work when suddenly a car jumps the curb and hits you, breaking your leg. As you writhe in pain, passersby don't stop to help but give you peculiar glances as if you were from another planet. Finally, the ambulance arrives, and the emergency medical technicians place you in the van on a stretcher. During this process, you catch one of them rolling his eyes as if you were faking the injury. On arrival at the emergency room, you have X-rays taken that confirm the diagnosis, and the doctor begins planning to take you into the operating room to repair your leg. But all the while, nurses, and even your family members, insinuate the accident was your fault and completely within your control. "Why didn't you know to get out of the way?" "What were you thinking?" "Come on, snap out of it. It can't hurt that bad." You would likely be appalled at the way you were being treated. How could you have anticipated the car jumping the curb and breaking your leg? And how could someone else know how bad the pain was?

Unfortunately, these types of reactions are exactly what individuals with mental illness experience almost on a daily basis. "Why don't you try not being depressed?" "It's all in your head. Just change the way you see things." "Well, lying around in the house isn't helping. You should do something else." None of these sound too consoling or supportive, but all too often, these are the types of reactions people with mental illness experience.

Statistically, about one-quarter of the population suffer from some type of mental health disturbance at some point in their lives. Of these millions, only one-quarter describe others as being compassionate about and empathetic with their problems. In other words, 75 percent of individuals with mental health disorders feel isolated, misunderstood, and/or ostracized for their conditions. Without question, a stigma surrounds mental health disorders and those suffering from these conditions, which contrasts greatly with perceptions of physical illnesses. When it comes to mental health conditions, people tend to assume individuals have greater levels of control simply because the symptoms and signs are less tangible. Can you imagine being treated that way if a car smashed into your leg?

While diagnostic tests for mental illnesses are not the same as they are for other medical conditions, psychiatric disorders do have a biological basis of causation. Genetic abnormalities, neurochemical imbalances, and altered neuroanatomy have all been attributed as causes for specific mental health disorders. Just because science and technology have yet to reveal all the details of how such disorders develop does not justify the view that individuals with mental health problems need to "just deal with their complaints." The explosion of new therapies, medications, and other treatments for a variety of psychiatric disturbances supports the fact that these conditions are really no different from other medical problems at a foundational level. As more advances are made, this fact will be increasingly evident.

For these reasons, mental health problems should not be feared or ignored. Individuals with psychiatric symptoms need attention and treatment, and you can help. Their conditions do not stem from a lack of willpower, an inherent mental weakness, or a failure to take charge of their lives. Instead, they suffer from a real, organic health problem that has affected their ability to emote, think, and function in a productive way. Regardless of whether an individual's condition involves a personality disorder, a mood disturbance, a perceptual condition, or some other mental health problem, they need proper diagnosis and care to overcome this difficulty. In many cases, they need support from friends and family while doing so.

From the preceding chapters, it should be evident that great hope exists in the care and treatment of mental health disorders. In some cases, medication breakthroughs have occurred, resulting in individuals being able to return to productive lives. Others benefit from various forms of therapy and counseling to a significant degree. In considering these options of care, a common theme often surfaces. Optimal mental health care requires prompt recognition and early treatment. All too often, because of the stigma previously described and a lack of knowledge about mental illness, individuals fail to receive diagnosis and care in an efficient manner. In some cases, a window of opportunity is missed, while in others a better quality of life is postponed. Through the information presented in this book, we have striven to highlight the importance of getting help early and the hope that comes from proper mental health care. Through instilling the principles of recovery and resiliency, individuals as well as families will be able to return to a functional state of health, while developing abilities to withstand future challenges.

While the information we have provided has been presented in a way to facilitate understanding of various categories of mental health, the individual chapters can be used as a reference when specific questions arise. We have provided additional resource links for a variety of subjects and conditions, which may serve to further your understanding and knowledge in specific areas (see Appendix). These same links offer support services, which may be quite valuable. Mental health care is an ever-evolving field with new discoveries and insights occurring all the time. Continuing to invest in a better understanding of these disorders can only serve to help you be a resource to those you care about the most.

Today, we live in a world that thrives on information. Those with information have power, while those who don't struggle. The same concept can be applied to mental health. Without knowledge of various mental health conditions, there is a lack of insight into how best to care for individuals suffering from psychiatric symptoms. Instead of recognizing warning signs, complaints are minimized or ignored. Our mission throughout this book has been to provide information so that you may have the knowledge necessary to help loved ones get the help they need. The knowledge you have gained provides you with the power to make a difference in their lives. Ultimately, this will have a positive impact on your life and for society at large.

Resources and Links

Mental Health Hotlines, Helplines, and Call Centers

Borderline Personality Disorder Resource Center: 1-888-694-2273
Information resource to assist with concerns about you or a loved one with possible BPD as well as phone counseling. http://www.bpdre-sourcecenter.org/

National Association of Anorexia Nervosa and Associated Disorders: 1-630-577-1330
National helpline for those suffering from eating disorders, with immediate counseling and treatment/support recommendations available. http://www.anad.org/eating-disorders-get-help/eating-disorders-helpline-email/

National Eating Disorder Association Helpline: 1-800-931-2237
Helpline staffed by trained individuals providing information about eating disorders, treatment options, and referrals for individuals with eating disorders. http://www.nationaleatingdisorders.org/information-referral-helpline/

National Sexual Assault Hotline: 1-800-656-4673
Hotline providing counseling and resource information for individuals who have been sexually assaulted. https://rainn.org/

National Suicide Prevention Hotline: 1-800-273-8255
A 24/7 support hotline staffed by skilled workers, and a mental health referral resource for individuals with suicidal thoughts and concerns. http://www.suicidepreventionlifeline.org/

Obsessive Compulsive Anonymous Nationwide Conference Call: 1-712-432-0075
Call center for individuals with OCD providing a twelve-step model to provide treatment through connection with peers. http://www .obsessive-compulsiveanonymous.org/

Samaritan's Crisis Hotline: 1-212-673-3000
A 24/7 suicide prevention hotline staffed by trained volunteers providing phone services, allowing individuals with suicidal thoughts to talk, express themselves, and be heard. http://samaritansnyc.org/24 -hour-crisis-hotline/

The Trevor Project: 1-866-488-7386
A national 24-hour, toll-free confidential suicide hotline for LGBTQ youth. http://www.thetrevorproject.org/

Mental Health Support Groups

American Foundation for Suicide Prevention—Offering support for victims of suicide loss as well as support for those at risk for suicide. http://afsp.org/find-support/ive-lost-someone/find-a-support-group/

Anxiety and Depression Association of America Support Groups—Support and resource lists provided for a variety of mood disturbances including anxiety, phobias, depression, relationship problems, and self-esteem issues. http://www.adaa.org/supportgroups

Co-Dependents Anonymous—A twelve-step program designed to empower individuals, eliminate self-destructive habits, and enhance self-esteem. http://coda.org/

Depression and Bipolar Support Alliance—Organization with more than seven hundred national peer-support groups to aid those with depression and bipolar disorder. http://www.dbsalliance.org/

Heal Grief—Nationwide grief support services organized state by state. http://healgrief.org/grief-support-resources/NATIONAL/

International OCD Foundation—Provides a listing of local OCD support groups internationally. https://iocdf.org/find-help/

National Alliance on Mental Illness—A grassroots mental health organization associated with hundreds of local affiliates, state organizations, and volunteers who work in the community to raise mental health awareness and provide support and education. https://www.nami .org/

National Association of Anorexia Nervosa and Associated Disorders—Various eating disorder support groups with psychotherapist and nutritionist support. http://www.anad.org/eating-disorders-get-help /eating-disorders-support-groups/

National Eating Disorders Association—Provides extensive list of local and regional support groups for various eating disorders and personalized peer-support locator services. http://www.nationaleatingdisorders .org/find-treatment/support-groups-research-studies

Postpartum Support International—Organization providing support, education, advocacy, and research for people living with mental illness in relation to pregnancy and postpartum periods. http://www .postpartum.net

Sidran's Help Desk—Services provided for all individuals suffering from PTSD as well as information about PTSD support groups. http://www.sidran.org/help-desk/get-help/

Addiction Support Groups

Al-Anon—Support services for individuals who have been affected by others' alcohol use and addiction. Also offers specialized programs for teenagers (Alateen). http://www.al-anon.org

Alcoholics Anonymous—Well-known program and support group for alcoholics with more than two million members internationally. http://www.aa.org

Cocaine Anonymous—Peer-support group and twelve-step program for individuals suffering from addiction to cocaine. http://www.ca.org

Crystal Meth Anonymous—Peer-support group and twelve-step program model for individuals struggling with addiction to crystal methamphetamine with more than six hundred meetings worldwide. http://www.crystalmeth.org

Dual Recovery Anonymous—A twelve-step program model designed for individuals with various chemical dependencies as well as emotional or psychological problems. Addresses both addiction and mood-related problems. http://draonline.qwknetllc.com/index.html

Gamblers Anonymous—Long-standing twelve-step program model for individuals struggling with gambling addiction. http://www.gamblers -anonymous.org/ga/locations/

LifeRing—Nonreligious organization providing forums and face-to-face meetings to aid individuals with addictions to design their own recovery plans. http://lifering.org

Marijuana Anonymous—National organization offering meetings and support for individuals struggling with marijuana addiction issues. https://www.marijuana-anonymous.org

Nar-Anon—Comparable to Al-Anon and Alateen in that this support program offers assistance to those affected by individuals with narcotic and other chemical dependencies. http://www.nar-anon.org /naranon/

Narcotics Anonymous—A peer-support program and twelve-step model to aid individuals with a variety of chemical addictions and dependencies, including narcotic medications. http://www.na.org

Overeaters Anonymous—Support group for individuals with food addictions with more than 6,500 meetings internationally. Program designed as a twelve-step model. http://www.oa.org

Sex Addicts Anonymous—Peer-support group and twelve-step model designed to assist those with sex-related addictions with meetings available internationally. https://saa-recovery.org

SMART Recovery—Alternative nonreligious support and treatment group for alcoholics and those with addictions that uses research-based cognitive behavioral therapies, with a focus on personal empowerment. http://www.smartrecovery.org

Women for Sobriety—Gender-specific, women-only support program to overcome chemical and alcohol addictions, using techniques to improve self-worth, personal responsibility, and problem-solving skills with locations in the US and Canada. http://www.womenfor -sobriety.org/beta2/

Index

Notes

Notes

Notes

Notes

Notes

Notes

Notes

....

....

....

....

....

....

....

....

....

....

....

....

....

....

Notes

Notes